'Robin Tipple gives a moving portrait of life in the long [...] Drawing on psychoanalysis, sociology and twentieth c[...] a historical record, a witness account, and a powerful theoretical analysis of the institutions of the late twentieth century. It is also a personal memoire that takes the reader on a journey, introducing two people whose lives were circumscribed by such an institution and who touched the author profoundly. The narrative account demonstrates vividly, and with deep compassion, how to listen to those whose words may, at first, seem to lack coherence. Based on notes made at the time, the story shows how meaning may evolve, and a relationship develop, through the medium of art psychotherapy. Thus, the book is relevant to therapists of today and will be of interest to arts therapists, counsellors and psychotherapists and all working with those who are marginalised. It will also inform researchers interested in the "total institutions" of the past and their residents'.

Professor Joy Schaverien, *PhD, Jungian psychoanalyst, art psychotherapist, author of* The Revealing Image *and* Boarding school Syndrome: The Psychological Trauma of the 'Privileged' Child

'This honest and engaging book includes two stories about the therapeutic relationships and imaginative lives of people with mild to moderate learning disabilities in a long-term institution. The book's details are pertinent to a broad range of therapeutic work but particularly consider the cultural expressions found in Art Therapy. The life stories described include the clients and the therapist (the author) because the autobiographic nature of much that is named "case study" is not evaded. The book interlaces events in the outside world with the internal psychological experiences of client and therapist. In this way, the book repeatedly returns to the theme of working-class identity and how it has shaped discourse certainly about the lives of people with learning disabilities but also the lives of many others. The book is important because it contributes to a discussion about how people caught up in institutional systems gain an internal sense of recognition from the other'.

Chris Wood, *PhD, NHS art therapist and research fellow, University of Sheffield*

'In times that seem increasingly concerned with swift and simple therapeutic solutions, Tipple's book offers something different and much needed: a detailed and reflective account of individual long-term Art Therapy with people with learning disabilities. Illuminating several single case narratives with thoughts from psychoanalysis, philosophy and Art Therapy, Tipple reminds us why it is important to muse on stories from therapy. Beyond giving evidence that Art Therapy is exceptionally suited for people marginalised for their cognitive impairment, he offers reflections on the human condition as such. Tipple's notion of therapy as a unique intersubjective process shows what Art Therapy can be: thoughtful, compassionate, respectful, dedicated and above all, deeply human'.

Uwe Herrmann, *PhD, professor on the MA programme in Art Therapy at Weissensee Academy of Art, Berlin*

'A necessary treasure in the shifting landscape of Art Therapy, research, and practice, with gently powerful rendering of a lifetime of reflective thinking, being and making in the field. The reader will benefit from Tipple's expressions of critical thinking around the stories notated, each "subject's" narrative offers thoughts on power dynamics, the materiality within relationship, and how the work lives in a reflexive clinical frame. Tipple highlights the continued necessity to think-through the subjective and intersubjective in relating, and to embed this in continued learning through research. His writings enlighten and provoke as he translates the human experience in the setting and context, time, and space, offering consideration of the philosophical and cultural in the pursuit of "linking", reciprocity, and personhood. He supports the reader to seek the in-between and engage with the wonderful possibilities within the alliance. This book is an essential read for every art therapist'.

Kristen Catchpole, *art psychotherapist who has worked with families, children, and vulnerable adults, lecturer at Goldsmiths University, London*

'Robin Tipple provides an original take on the Art Psychotherapy case study in contextualising therapy with two institutionalised patients in relation to his own life experience. His many years of practice, teaching and research in the learning disability field are apparent in the scope and depth of his reflections. He draws on the work of Sartre in making the case that, with time and consistency, a degree of mutual "recognition" within the therapeutic relationship is achievable. The value of paying close attention to gestures and mark making, as a physical manifestation of inner emotion, is also demonstrated in the two case studies. The prejudiced and elitist agendas that underpin the history of intelligence testing and learning disability diagnosis and treatment are succinctly analysed, and his account of the impact of institutional care on the lives of "Amy" and "Edward" serves as a timely reminder of the devastating emotional cost of an overly medicalised and behavioural approach to diagnosis, treatment, and care'.

Kim Dee, *art therapist, lecturer in Art Psychotherapy at Goldsmiths University, London, long previous experience as member of Community Learning Disability Service in Tower Hamlets*

Art Therapy in a Learning Disability Setting

This book originates from the experience of providing Art Therapy for adults diagnosed with learning disabilities living in an institutional setting. It follows two longitudinal case studies in an attempt to understand dyadic relations in Art Therapy.

Representing an important contribution to the history of Art Therapy, especially as it relates to the history of learning disabilities, this book explores past and contemporary discourses and contexts to identify a meaningful, thoughtful approach to the making and reading of images and the client/therapist relationship. It presents the thinking that informed the author's practice at the time, from both the point of view of the time and its present moment, to contextualize contemporary Art Therapy practice. Through the storytelling of long-term Art Therapy cases with thoughtful investigation, the author explores themes of melancholia, abjection, and alienation, while also creating a depth to current practice. The chapters are richly illustrated, the two case studies are personal and compelling, and the writing is accessible to all readers.

The book will appeal to practicing and training therapists of all persuasions, but especially those in Art Therapy or learning disability fields that have an interest in the visual forms of imagining and communicating.

Robin Tipple is an art therapist who has worked with adults and children in the NHS for 26 years and lectured at Goldsmiths, University of London, where he completed his PhD in 2011. He has published many papers on Art Therapy, in journals and as book contributions.

Art Therapy in a Learning Disability Setting

Subjectivity and Institutional Life

Robin Tipple

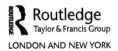

Routledge
Taylor & Francis Group

LONDON AND NEW YORK

Designed cover image: © *Metaphysical Portrait* by Robin Tipple

First published 2024
by Routledge
4 Park Square, Milton Park, Abingdon, Oxon OX14 4RN

and by Routledge
605 Third Avenue, New York, NY 10158

Routledge is an imprint of the Taylor & Francis Group, an informa business

British Library Cataloguing-in-Publication Data
A catalogue record for this book is available from the British Library

Library of Congress Cataloging-in-Publication Data
Names: Tipple, Robin, author.
Title: Art therapy in a learning disability setting: subjectivity and
institutional life / Robin Tipple.
Description: Abingdon, Oxon; New York, NY: Routledge, 2024. |
Includes bibliographical references and index. |
Identifiers: LCCN 2023037694 (print) | LCCN 2023037695 (ebook) |
ISBN 9781032418520 (hardback) | ISBN 9781032418513 (paperback) |
ISBN 9781003360056 (ebook)
Subjects: LCSH: Learning disabilities—Treatment—Case studies. |
Art therapy—Case studies. | Learning disabled—Mental health—Case
studies. | Learning disabled—Psychology—Case studies. | Learning
disabled—Means of communication—Case studies. | Visual
communication—Case studies.
Classification: LCC RC394.L37 T57 2024 (print) |
LCC RC394.L37 (ebook) | DDC 616.85/889—dc23/eng/20230927
LC record available at https://lccn.loc.gov/2023037694
LC ebook record available at https://lccn.loc.gov/2023037695

ISBN: 9781032418520 (hbk)
ISBN: 9781032418513 (pbk)
ISBN: 9781003360056 (ebk)

DOI: 10.4324/9781003360056

Typeset in Times New Roman
by codeMantra

Contents

Figures

Acknowledgements

I am, first, indebted to 'Amy' and 'Edward' (pseudonyms) and the residents of 'Hospital B' who allowed me to research and write about the work we did together; this included a presentation of their drawings and paintings. I was lucky in gaining the encouragement of Hospital Staff who advised me in relation to ethical considerations. I also benefitted greatly from the advice given by Dr Andrea Gilroy and Professor Diane Waller when writing up the two cases in this book for the MA in Art Psychotherapy. My practices improved, if at all, because I had an excellent clinical supervisor, Tessa Dalley, who also encouraged me to write. If this text has achieved some clarity, it is because of the perceptive and sensitive help provided by Chris Brown, who has always found time to do some reading for me, and he fully deserves my sincere gratitude. I would also like to thank Diana Velada and Dr Sally Skaife who have given their time to read through earlier drafts, both of whom have provided wise and cogent comments. Lastly, but by no means least, I should thank my partner Linda for her support and patience, especially when my mind was often 'elsewhere'.

Introduction

My impulse to write this book originated from the experience of providing Art Therapy for adults diagnosed with mild to moderate learning disabilities living in a large hospital, for People with Learning Difficulties. The type of institution that Goffman (1987) would call a 'total institution'. Essentially, it is two longitudinal Art Therapy case-studies, case studies, which attempt to represent inter-subjective processes as they emerged in the Art Therapy setting, mediated by the material element, chiefly the art materials and the products produced. The setting itself was shaped by the hospital, and subject to the power relations and discursive practices, that are reproduced in total institutions.

I want to begin this book with the ontological claim that subjects exist, at least bodily, but also in the form of persons, referred to or represented, in a text or a practice. Like others, I suspect, I think of persons as human, capable of actions, and of experiencing the world, material and social, which implies being for others. I also prefer to think of subjects as always in the process of becoming. This becoming other, through relationship, is where the debate begins perhaps, where the problems of identifying subjects, subjectivity and inter-subjectivity, emerges.

The book is a re-iteration in the sense that it revisits some previous writing which was submitted as an academic assignment on a master's course in 1995. This writing has not been previously published, and for this book, it has been comprehensively edited and rewritten, using later insights gained from PhD and post-doctoral research. Because I am attempting to address problems that I dimly recognised previously, but developed inadequately, my hope is that the re-iteration, with additional material which makes use of my own subsequent researches, experiences and reflections, will offer fresh insight. What I believe I have to offer is related to a particular way of working in Art Therapy, which has its roots in psychoanalytical object relations theory, but which has been developed in practice, through an engagement with other philosophical and cultural literatures. This book should be of interest to all art therapists, not just therapists working with the Learning Disabled, in that it provides two detailed longitudinal studies of contexts, therapeutic relations, and Art production in Art Therapy, which enables thought in relation to subjectivity and intersubjectivity in an institutional setting to emerge.

DOI: 10.4324/9781003360056-1

In 2010 the United States Senate passed a law called Rosa's Law to remove the term 'mental retardation' from use in official documentation and research journals and to replace it with Intellectual Disability. Intellectual Disability appears in the Diagnostic Statistical Manual of Mental Disorders 5th Edition published by the American Psychiatric Association 2013 under the broader heading of Neurodevelopmental Disorders. Intellectual Developmental Disorders is the term used by the International Classification of Diseases 11th Edition, published by the World Health Organisation 2018. Both diagnostic manuals stress 'deficits in general mental ability' which appear when the 'individual fails to meet expected developmental milestones' in 'several areas' of functioning (DSM V 2013, p31). Development is usually assessed via a clinical observation which is framed by an agreement in relation to normality. Such an assessment would seek support from physical examinations and medical examinations and a confirmation of diagnosis from the administration of standardised intelligence tests.

Intellectual Disabilities are categorised according to IQ levels achieved on standardised intelligence tests; 50–70 mild, 35–50 moderate, 20–35 severe, and below 20 profound. However, DSM V does suggest that the levels of severity should be 'defined on the basis of adaptive functioning, and not IQ scores, because it is adaptive functioning that determines the level of supports required' and also that 'IQ measures are less valid in the lower end of the IQ range' (DSM V 2013, p33).

I shall use the term People with Learning Disabilities in this book to refer to people diagnosed with 'Intellectual Disability' as this is the preferred term of the people themselves. I prefer 'disability' to 'difficulties' as there are many different forms of discreet learning difficulties that do not have the more *general* character of a disability of the kind that is regarded as present in Learning Disability. Most labels in this diagnostic domain have a pejorative feel, and it is difficult to escape this. Neuro-diversity might be a way out of this difficulty, but it doesn't necessarily help us differentiate between impairments, if, and when, they are identified, and disabilities which are more social in origin.

As I have indicated above, this book is about People with Learning Disabilities who have been diagnosed as having a Mild to Moderate disability, subjects who had been living in a large hospital for most of their adult life. In this situation it is very difficult to be sure of impairment and disability. I should add here that large institutions, like Hospital B which this book is describing, no longer exist, although many people with learning disabilities do still live institutional lives that are restricted in terms of opportunity and relationship. For a discussion of the relation between impairment and disability see Slorach (2016, p67–p69).

Chapter 1 considers in more detail the discourses that are present in DSM V and inform the construction of practices which identify the learning disabled. These are identified above, they are, namely medical discourses as they reference physical and neurological abnormality, developmental discourses – especially those concerned with psychological development, and the discourses that identify intelligence and are productive of intelligence testing. Discourses are of interest to me throughout this book and I adopted a broad definition which includes 'language in use, as a process which is socially situated'. It encompasses 'written discourse' which structures 'areas of knowledge and the social and institutional practices which are associated with them'. In so far as discourses are productive in relation to 'worlds', they reproduce and construct 'afresh' practices that are 'constrained or encouraged' by larger movements in the social, cultural and political environment (see Candlin 1997, pix).

I give more weight to the history of intelligence testing than developmental discourses or medical discourses, in Chapter 1, as this helps us in our thinking about the way in which intelligence and mind has been identified and located in psychological and scientific discourses. These are discourses which are engaged in the search for measures, which can produce the confirmation for the existence of an impairment. The chapter ends with a brief, more alternative consideration of where we might locate mind.

In Chapter 2, I explore the use of case study in Art Therapy researches. This could be regarded as a problematic area of research, but I try to show why it is important for art therapists to continue to produce case studies, and in support of this, I include in this chapter some account of the development of my own thinking, made possible by researching the work I was engaged in. Case studies are directed towards the description of 'subjects' and they depend on the therapist's appreciation of 'subjectivity'.

There are two parts to Chapter 3. In Part 1, I will be providing the reader with some brief narratives constructed from my remembered past, autobiographical fragments that focus on childhood, adolescence, a working life begun in the Royal Air Force, and my experiences at Art School and University. I have tried to identify my responses to the demands of new situations, as I progressed through early adulthood. I want to show how I was shaped by, and how I reacted to institutional life, and disciplinary practices. My brief account of Art School and University years which have shaped my current commitment to art production, and interest in class relations and social justice, ends Part 1.

Part 2 of this chapter presents Hospital 'B' and the Art Therapy Department. In constructing my account of hospital 'B', I have examined a small illustrated booklet presented to the public as 'Hospital History', produced by the hospital at the moment of its official closure. This is not fully referenced, as I wish to maintain hospital anonymity. The booklet gives some account of the hospital's organisation, as manifest in its spatial arrangements and its material facilities. This information has been supplemented by a literature research and personal recollection. My aim is to present a picture of changing practices and discourses that shaped life for the patients/residents and those that worked in Hospital B.

The case studies, in Chapters 4 and 5, constitute the justification for this book. The studies include an examination of communication in detail, as far as my notes, and the illustrations, allow, facilitating some access to the hermeneutic problem of the art work and the problematic of the voice, which are linked (see Skaife 2000).

I have tried to present something of the emotional impact of the work, on both the therapist and hospital resident in the writing, and I have also given attention to the implications of the physical and discursive environment, including power relations, as they affected the therapeutic relationship over time. I wanted to capture something of the character of the intersubjective exchanges that were central to the possibility of thought and creativity.

Amy appears in Chapter 4. She began her Art Therapy at 62 years of age. She was born with Spina Bifida and was thought to have mild to moderate learning disabilities. Amy had lived in hospital B for 45 years, before I met her. We met weekly for 64 weeks.

Chapter 5 presents the second of my two cases, Edward, a 50 year old man, who was also diagnosed as having mild to moderate learning disabilities, but in addition, mental health problems (schizophrenia). Edward had lived in hospital B for 34 years. Edward attended Art Therapy for just under six years, and we met on a weekly basis.

The book ends with a concluding speculative discussion focussed on recognition. Here I make use of Hegel, Butler and Sartre, in conceptualising recognition and in placing recognition within Hospital B, and the case material that I have been exploring. I also try to show briefly how recognition was important for both the resident, and the art therapist (myself), in enabling reciprocity to establish relationship in the art therapy Process.

References

Candlin, C. N. 1997. General Editors Preface. In: Gunnarsson, B. L., Linnell, P. & Nordberg, B. (Eds.) *The Construction of Professional Discourse.* Longman, London, pp. ix–xiv.

DSM V. 2013. *Diagnostic and Statistical Manual of Mental Disorders.* American Psychiatric Association, Washington, D.C.

Goffman, E. 1987. *Asylums – Essays on the Social Situation of Mental Patients and Other Inmates.* Peregrine Books – Penguin Books, London.

Skaife, S. 2000. Keeping the Balance: Further Thoughts on the Dialectics of Art Therapy, Chapter 5. In: Gilroy, A. & McNeilly, G. (Eds.) *The Changing Shape of Art Therapy – New Developments in Theory and Practice.* Jessica Kingsley Publishers, London, Philadelphia, pp. 115–142.

Slorach, R. 2016. *A Very Capitalist Condition – A History and Politics of Disability.* Bookmarks Publications, London.

Chapter 1

Mind and Three Discursive Domains

In this chapter, I want to explore some elements from the three discursive domains that were identified in the introduction as productive in diagnostic practices when identifying neuro-developmental disorders (see DSM V), namely medical discourses, developmental discourses and intelligence testing. I am focussing on those elements in the discourses that are aimed at the identification of mind and intelligence. I want to know how mind and intelligence have been characterised, represented, disclosed and measured. This has importance in relation to the hospital residents who appear as subjects in my two case studies.

Amy and Edward were diagnosed as having mild to moderate Learning Disabilities. In the DSM V, this would be called mild to moderate Intellectual Disability. When Amy and Edward were incarcerated in Hospital B in early adolescence a 'deficit' in intelligence was suspected, the diagnosis then in use would have been 'defective', 'imbecile' or 'feeble-minded', but no standardised measure was undertaken until late in their lives after having been confined in the institution for some years. Amy was tested after she had been in the hospital for 37 years, and Edward was tested after 18 years in the hospital. It is Amy's and Edward's mind that is in question, and having a diagnosis that claims to have identified an impairment in mental capacity, applied to one, results in a response from the other. At the end of this chapter, I present some thinking in relation to the location of mind.

Medical Discourses

Foucault in *The Birth of the Clinic* sought to interrogate the conditions for the 'possibility of medical experience' (Foucault 2003, pxxii). He endeavours to show us how the nature of language and reason is related to the Medical gaze. The Doctor 'in order to know ... must recognize while already being in possession of the knowledge that will lend support to his recognition' (p9). The first task, in France at least at the end of the 18th century, was to recognise health. Foucault argued that 'one did not think first of the internal structure of *the organized being,* but of *the medical polarity of the normal and the pathological*' (emphasis in the original, p41).

If the disease presents itself to the attentive Doctor through experience, if it is manifest to the attentive and free gaze, it is not initially speakable or open to

DOI: 10.4324/9781003360056-2

language. To address this issue, it becomes necessary to establish 'a structured no-sological field' where 'different diseases serve as the text' (p70). 'The patient is the *subject* of his disease ... the patient is the accident of his disease, the transitory object that it happens to have seized upon' (emphasis in original, p71). For Foucault, it is the nosological, the tabulation of agreed diseases, not unlike the DSM, which allows for language to develop in relation to the medical gaze. What is revealed is 'the tangible space of the body, which at the same time is that opaque mass in which secrets, ... the very mystery of origins lie hidden' (p150).

In the clinic, inquiry was aimed at establishing the history and progress of a disease, and the links between symptoms. Corpses were dissected principally for educating surgeons, and it was some while before pathological anatomy could be understood as capable of revealing disease. It first became necessary for physicians to interrogate anatomical space, to create a geography in relation to the clinic's account of chronologies and symptoms. What is discovered in pathological anatomy is that disease, life and death are bound together, disease as 'that possibility internal to life' and where 'Death', also internal to life, thereby becomes a possibility, 'it is because he may die that a man falls ill', in life (p191). 'Degeneration' then becomes a matter of concern, 'That weakening of natural robust humanity'. 'In this notion', Foucault suggests, 'is gathered up all that was most negative in the historical, the atypical, and the counter-natural' (p192). It is essentially the discovery of death, in life, that enables the medical gaze to be both 'spatialized and individualized' in the, malformations, lesions, tissues and textures of the body, to be examined and compared, one case with another.

The idea of 'Degeneracy' brings with it at the end of the 19th century a fear of that 'indefinite and confused family of 'abnormals''. Discursive domains that reveal the 'abnormals', Foucault argues, were 'formed' from three elements; 'The human monster'; 'The individual to be corrected'; and 'The onanist'. The human monster is conceived of as a 'natural' deviation from 'nature', and the doctor is asked 'is this individual dangerous?', here there are uncertainties. The individual to be corrected 'is a more recent figure than the monster'. What then emerges is the notion of the 'incorrigible' which requires institutions of confinement and correction. The 'onanist' appears 'in connection with new relations between sexuality and the family organisation' (Foucault 2000, p52 & p53), here importance is given to the body and to health, and the discipline that is necessary to defend society.

These 'fears' identified by Foucault do provide some further explanation for the anxieties of the Eugenicists at the beginning of the 20th century; their interest in morality; their desire to ensure the continuous production of a healthy population; and their desire to protect the status quo.

Tredgold (1908) established four categories of 'defectives', as people with learning disabilities, and others whose mentality was in question, were then named:

a Idiots – 'deeply defective' who are 'unable to guard themselves against common physical dangers'
b Imbeciles – a defectiveness that does not amount to idiocy but the individual is 'incapable of managing themselves' and is unable to be taught how to do so.

c Feeble-minded persons 'whose weakness' does not amount to imbecility yet they require care and cannot benefit from instruction.
d Moral-imbeciles who exhibit 'vicious or criminal propensities' and do not respond to punishment.

In his identification of 'Amentia' (the absence of mind) Tredgold stressed that the 'normal mind' has a 'degree of intellectual capacity' that enables the performance '*of duties as a member of society in that position of life to which he was born*' (p2, italics in the original). In Tredgold, we can see that the 'defective' becomes an individual unable to assume his or her predetermined social role, incorrigible when unable to 'benefit from instruction', and perhaps a 'monster' or 'onanist' when we consider the 'moral imbecile', whose absence of mind, or degree of imperfection of mind, is exhibited in his or her 'vicious or criminal propensities'.

As nosology developed and expanded, doctors who were concerned about a suspected lack of development and intellectual ability, focussed on the body, from both the external and internal perspective, and the increase in instrumental examinations lead to the identification of 'malformation' through comparisons and the collection of specimens. Contemporary researches and diagnostic procedures can make use of prenatal ultrasounds, X rays, and MRI, all productive of imagery which can be collated with the analysis of cells and post-mortem findings and case records. To enable recognition to take place, clinicians will consult the contemporary record, the current pictorial Atlas being the *Atlas of Genetic Diagnosis and Counselling – 3rd Edition –* Chen (2017). Two hundred and ninety identified genetic diseases and malformations are illustrated and presented by colour photography, in the atlas. In support of the photography, there are descriptions of 'malform' (the shorthand for malformation), an account of the diseases' genetics, the diagnostic tests in use, which include cytogenetic, biochemical and molecular techniques. This nosology also provides case presentations, which illustrate the course of individual diseases and a history of the patients' family.

In the clinic setting teams are now organised to produce a diagnostic assessment. They may be organised according to democratic ideals that allow for different perspectives to be included in discussions. David Henley the art therapist gives a good account of this approach to diagnosis. He provides a case by way of example. The 'team leader, a neuropsychologist', began the discussion of the case, the subject being a deaf child, by referencing 'neuro-hormonal and cognitive deficits'. The child's teacher pointed to language difficulties, and the social worker to mother's 'marked lack of warmth', while 'a minority team member' argued that the mother's behaviour was indicative of 'a cultural difference' rather than pathology. What Henley's description shows is that team discussions became 'more contentious and personalised' when cultural or political issues arose in the situation, and overall it is 'genetics and neuroscience' that holds 'sway over those [team members] oriented within the withering humanities' (Henley 2012, p50 & p52).

Medical science then would appear to emphasise that picture of the mind that presents brain and mind as synonymous, where behaviour is regarded as a peripheral result. Nevertheless, impairment is still viewed as having a presence in adaptive functioning, that is, in a failure of the person's effectiveness in meeting the social expectations for his or her age, by his or her cultural group, a failure in relation to 'duty' in Tredgold's language. But the discourse does not allow for any sustained study of social expectations and the cultural group, since brain and mind are indissolubly linked to genetic inheritance, and all that is required is to investigate the genetics of the case and discover, where that is possible, what takes place at a neurological level. It is, to transport Foucault's (2003, p150) words to a more contemporary context, in the 'tangible space' of the brain that 'the very mystery of origins lie hidden' for neurologists.

Development

Developmental theory, in relation to the human, is predicated on the differences between the adult and the child. Childhood is perceived as 'natural' and we assume the child to be lacking in the rationality of the adult. We were all children after all and mistaken, unacquainted with the world. Nevertheless, it is thought, we grow and develop into adulthood. This might be the view which belongs to folk-psychology. Jenks argues that childhood is 'spoken about as: a 'becoming'; as a 'laying down [of] the foundations;' as 'growing up;...' There is, he points out, an essential relation to 'an unexplicated, but nevertheless firmly established, rational adult world' (Jenks 1996, p9).

Jenks tells us that childhood is not the same everywhere; it emerges from the 'structuring of social relations', from 'organizations of family life, ideologies of care and philosophies of need and dependency'. We should note that the discourses that are productive in respect of childhood and children 'do not have an equivalence'. They are 'arranged hierarchically'. The 'child-discourse of social workers or juvenile magistrates have a power and efficacy in excess of those of the sibling or parent,' for instance. Discourses 'derive from the dominant cultural image of the 'normal' child' and the child exists 'within a network of relations, a matrix of partial interests and a complex of forms of professional knowledge, that are beyond the physical experience of being a child' (Jenks 1996, p69).

Whilst Jenks alerts us to the social and the cultural in relation to childhood, the study of childhood in relation to mind could be said to begin in the 1840s with Darwin. Darwin was in search of the 'origins and specificities of mind – the human adult mind.' Inheritance and environment was emphasised and the child was seen as 'repeating evolutionary process in its own developmental trajectory'. According to Berman's (2017) account of the history of Developmental Psychology, the 'newly discovered' mental life of the child was 'a subjectivity' accorded to 'the middle-class child' – whereas the depraved 'children of the poor' were regarded as animal and primitive. Women were also thought to be closer to 'children and primitives' in terms of competence and maturity (see Burman 2017, p15, p16 & p18).

These early studies established the direction of developmental research. The mind was 'conceived of as singular, separate but universal'. It was 'instantiated' in the development of the minds of children, the assumption being that 'there is a normal core of development unfolding according to biological principles'. The studies produced a split between 'emotion and rationality' which emerged in the practice of the research, this is later reflected in the 'complementary relation between psychology and psychoanalysis' (Burman 2017, p19).

In Victorian England 'the poor health of army recruits' and the establishment of compulsory elementary schooling 'generated anxieties about 'pauperism' which was viewed as a 'trait rather than a set of circumstances'. The 'feeble-minded' in this climate 'came to signify physical, moral, mental and political disintegration' (Burman 2017, p20) comments, and we can see this is in the Mental Deficiency Act (1913). 'Individual psychology' emerged to enable classification and surveillance of a population, which became possible in the school, in hospitals, in clinics and in the army. The mental qualities of individuals could be compared with the general population, the insane could be divided from the sane and 'educable from the ineducable'. Thus the development and evaluation of mental testing is required (Burman 2017, p19 & p21). Widespread mental testing produces, through the use of statistics, norms – as we shall see when we consider the history intelligence testing in more detail in this chapter.

Behaviourist ideas impacted on developmental psychology 'from the 1910s onward', and they gave emphasis to the environment, to 'school as well as family' where training or 'education of the child and the parents' was intended to 'compensate' for the 'deficiencies of heredity'. This approach *gradually* 'superseded segregation', but it did require 'a commitment to greater intervention and control'. Control was evident in the 1930s, for example in Pintner (1933). Pinter writes in relation to the 'feeble minded':

'Since feeblemindedness is not a disease that we can hope to cure, what methods are to be adopted to lessen the enormous burden that feeblemindedness places on the community? The only procedures seem to be training, segregation and sterilization'.

... 'The segregation of feebleminded women of child bearing age is particularly necessary ... Perhaps the percentage is increasing in view of the very noticeable modern trend among the more intelligent families to limit the number of offspring, with little corresponding limitation among the less intelligent families'.

Pintner (1933, p837)

This agitation for sterilisation was particularly active in the 1930s; however, Burman (2017, p21) suggests that such 'sentiments' that align intelligence to class position, 'are still at play today'.

In 1950, the American Psychologist Arnold Gesell promoted the notion of development as a 'natural unfolding' that could be equated with growth, he sought to establish norms as 'milestones'. He was in favour of 'clinical interviews' rather than psychometric tests. His representations of development are 'age graded', for example they show that a child at 24 months, can build a tower of six or seven cubes, can fill a cup with cubes and hand it to the examiner. The 'mental is incorporated within the medical' in Gessell's account (Burman 2017, p23). Nurseries were designed to allow child observation, photography began to be used, common behaviours were documented, and the average achieves the status of the norm. Gessell does not tell us much about mind but he does establish the idea of the 'natural' which is firmly linked to the normal. But the natural is also productive of disease which can be seen in behaviour, when it deviates from the mean.

Piaget's descriptions of children's thinking, his 'genetic epistemology', became a popular replacement for behaviourism which had presented learning as entirely environmentally driven. Piaget presented children as actively constructing their learning environments. He emphasised adaptation. Particular forms of rationality can be encountered in Piaget who defines Developmental Psychology as 'the study of the development of mental functions'. Like Darwin he was in search of a 'complete description' of 'mind' in its 'finished state' (Piaget 1972, p72). Piaget's theories in relation to intelligence and child development presents intellectual development as staged, in early infancy 'sensory-motor' explorations; followed by 'pre-conceptual' thought; 'intuitive' thinking, 'concrete' operations, and finally, in early adolescence, 'formal operations'. Stages are, as we might expect, not only chronologically ordered but also given in a linear hierarchical form, from the infantile to adult 'operative intelligence'. Jenks argues that this 'sets a narrative in the discourse of cognitive growth that is by now global and overwhelming'. 'Operative intelligence is the providence of adulthood. It implies the informed manipulation and transformation of objects by a reflecting subject' (Jenks 1996, p24). It is an ideal exemplifying logical process. Logic epitomises modern scientific method and Piaget depicts the child as a 'budding scientist encountering problems in the material world, developing hypotheses and learning by discovery and activity'. This depiction 'treats the individual as prior and separate – qualities which also carry colonial and gendered nuances' argues Burman (2017, p244). This can be seen when the developing child becomes a boy in the advertising for 'educational toys' – 'He's researching surface texture, differentiating between colours, and developing his audio-sensory perception. He thinks he is playing with a rattle' (for Duplo in *Parents Magazine*, December 1984 – see Burman 2017, p244).

Piaget produces an account of the mind that stresses internal representations and abstraction leading to hypotheses prior to action. Archard (1993) argued that Piaget's 'ideal of adult cognitive competence is a peculiarly Western philosophical one.' 'If adult cognitive competence is conceived in this way then there is no reason to think it conforms to the everyday abilities of even Western adults' (Archard 1993, p65 & p66).

The Russian Developmental Psychologist Vygotsky was critical of Piaget, for neglecting language and culture, but he was supportive, in respect of Piaget's methodology. Vygotsky viewed developmental research as a form of teaching and as a 'practical promotion of children's psychological functioning in future situations'. In the context of any study the experimenter becomes an active participant, and, as with Piaget, the 'dependent variable'. In the British and US adaptations of Piaget, variables in the testing or experimental situation are all located in the child, and the context of the investigation is regarded 'as neutral or invisible' (Burman 2017, p240). In this model, there is no room for the examiners as variables.

This question in relation to the examiners is raised in Developmental Psychology when the social makes an appearance with 'Theory of Mind' (TOM). TOM represents the social in a reduced dyadic form, when considered in relation to interaction and communication, and is used to explicate a hypothesised failure in the understanding of other minds, a failure regarded as present in Autism. Here we can see that the experimental situation, which involves the child in identifying a 'false belief', provides a paradigm for 'the researchers, not just in the sense of procedure for testing knowledge of other minds in children, but as a tacit model of what making sense of other people must entail' (Leudar et al. 2004, p578). It produces a particular vision of mind: 'Both the idea that understanding requires a theory, and the idea that the theory is about other minds.' This reproduces 'the Cartesian assumption of one individual mind looking out at external reality to represent it as truthfully as possible' (Nelson et al. 2000). Bradley (1991) goes further than Nelson et al., and suggests that the experimental psychologist is promoting an 'illusory and idealized self-identity as – like anyone else who is 'normal' [he or she is] naturally immune from fantasy and unproblematically able to deduce the mental state of others' (Bradley 1991, p54).

TOM emerges from a Cognitive Psychology that seeks to identify a cognitive deficit which can be related to identifiable neurological functioning and thereby disclose an impairment. For instance, a malfunction in the mirror neuro system (MNS) was thought to be responsible for mind-blindness (Gallese and Goldman 1998), but this view was challenged by Fan et al. (2010) who were able to show that MNS was often 'relatively well preserved' in individuals who failed the TOM test. We should note here that individuals who pass the TOM test can still do badly in live situations where recognition of others in respect of mind is wanted, and vice versa, those who fail the TOM test can do well in vivo.

Cognitive psychologists themselves are not in total agreement in relation to TOM. Bruner and Feldman (1993) argue for the importance of early learning in respect of culturally mediated semiotic structures, and Hobson (1993) and Trevarthen et al. (1996) emphasise affect, and the recognition of feeling in understanding others. However, TOM has maintained its dominant position in this debate. Maybe because TOM is the kind of theory that supports Cognitive Psychology in its alignment with medical science, in promoting neurological primacy, and that which is inherited in respect of minds, it also supports Piaget's account of mind which emphasises logical operations, which represents the preferred intellectualist view of mind and epistemology.

Emotion does find a place within developmental discourses, but its contribution to thought is diminished and transformed into logically operative cognitive functions, which are supported by internal representations. Attachment Theory begins with love and hate (see Suttie 1988 (1935) pp xv–xviii). It is formed from the confluence of psychoanalysis, ethology, systems theory, and later evolutionary theory and neurology. It begins with the observation of children in a set situation. As some readers will know, mother takes her infant to a strange place and after a short period, she then leaves the child with a stranger who enters the space, and later she returns to reunite herself with the child. The observer is concerned to notice the child's emotional reactions, the objective being to determine if the child is ambivalent or avoidant in relation to his or her attachment to mother. This might be indicated by the child's inability to play at a distance from mother in the strange place, or a failure to protest when mother departs. But the important observation takes place when mother returns, and it is anticipated that a securely attached child would greet his mother with relief, perhaps enthusiastically, or angrily, but this could be an occasion when ambivalent or avoidant behaviour is more directly displayed. The theory becomes shaped later through the introduction of longitudinal studies of older children, interviews with caregivers (usually mothers), plus the development of an Adult Attachment Interview.

Mothers are required to demonstrate the presence of 'Emotional Availability' (E.A.) and 'Maternal Mindedness' (M.M.) in the attachment paradigm. Fonagy (2003a, 2003b), a later psychoanalytic researcher, argues that the 'mother's empathic emotion provides the infant with feedback on his emotional state. Thus 'the infant develops a secondary representation of his emotional state, with the mother's empathic face as the signifier and his own emotional arousal as the signified.' He goes on to say

> the contingent responding of the attachment figure is thus far more than the provision of reassurance ... it is the principal means by which we acquire understanding of our own internal states, which is an intermediate step in the acquisition of the understanding of others as psychological entities.
>
> Fonagy (2003a, p115 & p116)

The environment of the 'early relationship' with the caregiver is regarded as 'crucial' not necessarily in terms of future relationships but, Fonagy asserts, because it equips 'the individual with a mental processing system that will subsequently generate mental representations, including relationship representations' (Fonagy 2001, p31). We are back to an emphasis on particular discreet cognitive operations, the mental processing of internal representations, which we saw in TOM, which determines social response, and recognition of others. Attachment theory as developed by Fonagy (2003b) is also linked to neuroscience:

> 'Mothers were asked to respond to sad or smiling faces of their babies while in an fMRI scanner ... teenage mothers hardly differentiated between these two emotions in their infants' whereas 'the control women showed dramatic activation of the prefontal cortex (mPFC) and cingulated cortex, areas involved in emotion recognition and processing.' ... Teenage mothers, perhaps one of the highest risks groups for the disorganisation of attachment processes with their

children, appear to show a dramatic lack of differentiation for emotional displays in their infants.

Fonagy (2003b, p7)

As Burman points out emotions become 'a mere subsystem of cognition' (Burman 2017, p160) and Fonagy, having, seemingly, lost his links with psychoanalysis, which emphasises the uncertain nature of communication and relationship, gives a cognitive account of attachment which can be linked to neurology. The image of the mind that Fonagy supplies us with replicates that seen in TOM, where a behavioural pattern is linked to a hypothesised mental mechanism, the mental mechanism is then linked to neural activity, in a causal chain. The neural activity in TOM is named as the mirror neuro system (MNS), in attachment it becomes a system which includes the amygdala, pre-frontal cortex and the limbic system, or activity 'in the region of the insula' (Fonagy 2001, p46, 2003b, p7). This mind can be located in internal brain activity, it is rational and accessible to 'normal' adults. In this model, mentation, or thinking, is seen as abstracting information and hypothesising – in the manner of Piaget. Cultural tools, social pressures, desires, emotions and the transmission of affect, as problems to be researched, appear to have been lost, are now of peripheral interest.

O'Connor and Joffe (2013) comment, in relation to the researches on attachment, that women, as mothers, are presented in terms of 'good versus bad development, with middle-class full-time mothers objectifying the good and their working or working-class counterparts the bad' (p305). The working class, of course, have been presented in medical discourses, and some developmental discourses, as inheriting incapacities and impairments in relation to social adaptation and cognitive operations, as genetically lacking in intelligence. But how do we measure intelligence?

Intelligence and the Testing of Intelligence

Gould (1992) has produced a detailed and critical account of the history of intelligence testing. His history begins in the 19th century and ends in the late 1970s. I shall quote extensively from Gould's book in what follows, since the book describes clearly the social, cultural and political pressures that shaped modern approaches to intelligence and the practices of testing for intelligence that developed in America and Europe.

The beginnings can be regarded as a search for that 'thing in the head' which, in particular, would disclose racial differences, differences that were regarded as confirmation of the inevitability of European ascendency, and, it should not be forgotten, the *natural* superiority of man in relation to woman (Gould 1992, p23). As the brain was assumed to be 'the seat of mentality', it was thought that 'intelligence must reside there'.

The measure of intelligence began with the study of brain sizes and the measurement of skulls (craniometry). Morton, S. G. in his Crania Americana of 1839 presented his findings, his measurements of skulls, in a table that ranked human beings in hierarchically differentiated groups, the Teutonic Family, with the largest skulls, at the top and the Negro Group, whose skull sizes were presented, *erroneously*, as on average, smaller, at the bottom. This table, and ranking, was only possible because smaller samples from the Teutonic Family were removed, and averages overall were not properly calculated (see Gould 1992, p54). What was required by Morton, from the research, was found.

There was at the beginning a strong desire, amongst the scientific community, to 'assign all individuals to their proper status' through the production of 'an objective number' (Gould 1992, p24). Broca, P. writing from 1861 to 1876 in France, measured the volume within skulls. Like others measuring skulls he argued for the natural superiority of the European upper class Male but, as Gould argues, he was 'defeated' by his numbers, especially when measuring a large sample of skulls from Paris cemeteries. In his later researches, Broca included the measurement of frontal (anterior) regions and posterior regions of the skull and the measurement of the length of the skull and facial angle. But, whatever the measure or number achieved, Broca, through convoluted interpretations, continued to argue for his initial prejudice.

The assumptions, and prejudices, of the craniometrists decayed surprisingly slowly. Epstein, H. T. in 1978, for example, revived that initial investigation of intelligence that previously sought to link intelligence to the shape and the size of the head. He also argued for the natural inherent disadvantage, and advantage, of particular groups, and proposed that head sizes could be ordered in relation to vocational status. In his support, he provided a statistical correlation that brain size conferred an advantage. But this was another argument that was built on corrupted data and the statistical correlation that Eptstein references is so small as to lack any meaningful significance. As Gould shows, variation in brain size remains entirely independent of vocational status, or class.

Alfred Binet, director of the Psychology laboratory at the Sorbonne Publishing 1898–1916, wanted to measure the intelligence of school children and began his career by measuring heads. But he recognised an unconscious bias in his measurements and found that the differences between students in head sizes were very small and bore no relation to the intelligence exhibited by the students. So in 1904, Binet changed his technique and constructed tests. His task was to identify children who, failing in the classroom, may be in need of some form of special education. He wrote in 1911 'it matters little what the tests are so long as they are numerous' (Binet and Simon 1939, p329).

Binet arranged the tests according to their difficulty and assigned an age level. He tasked the children with completing the tests, and for the youngest to continue until they could no longer complete the tests. The 'age associated with the last test' that a subject child could complete became his 'mental age'. Initially, the child's intellectual level was determined by subtracting this mental age from his true age; however, 'in 1912, the German psychologist W. Stern argued that mental age should be divided by chronological age'. This would give the 'relative as opposed to the absolute' disparity between mental and chronological ages. So IQ was born (see Gould 1992, p149 & p150). Binet saw IQ as a rough guide, because he argued 'intelligence is not a single, scalable thing like height' [Binet and Simon 1939 (1911)]. He was clear that IQ was not to be understood as 'inborn intelligence', not to be seen as a mechanism for 'ranking all pupils according to mental worth'; but it was thought that it might have a value in identifying pupils needing 'special help' (Gould 1992, p152).

American psychologists were impressed with Binet's work, but they 'reified Binet's scores, and took them as measures of an entity called intelligence'. They argued that this 'intelligence was largely inherited' and not subject to change (Gould 1992, p157). Goddard (1914) developed a taxonomy. First there were 'idiots' – those incapable of the development of speech. These would be regarded today as having severe to profound intellectual disabilities, the group most difficult to test. Next in this linear grading comes 'imbeciles' – those incapable of mastering written language, those today regarded as having moderate intellectual disabilities. Finally we come to the 'feeble-minded' who Goddard choose to call 'morons' from the Greek word meaning foolish; this group were represented by IQs 50–70, moderate to mild intellectual disabilities in DSM V.

Goddard was concerned that 'morons', sometimes referred to as 'high-grade defectives', should be prevented from breeding to preserve the American stock; 'intelligent men rule in comfort and by right' and 'the people who are doing the drudgery ... are as a rule in their proper places' he claimed (Goddard 1919, p246). When measuring the IQ levels of immigrants, Goddard, assumed that those travelling third class to America were, on average, unintelligent 'morons', and the results of his testing confirmed this. This is not surprising since Goddard's assistants were selecting subjects, only from the third class or steerage, most of whom could speak little English and knew little of American life. They were tested immediately as they embarked. To confound the measures, Goddard's translation of Binet's tests scored people harshly.

Interestingly, Goddard in 1928 shifted, a little, in his view. He conceded that his tests had overestimated the number of 'feeble-minded', and he agreed with Binet that education could make a difference in the ability of 'morons' to 'manage themselves' (Goddard 1928, p220).

Terman (1919) used Binet's tests to create the Stanford-Binet test in 1919. There were 90 tasks in this test and it became the standard for 'virtually all' IQ tests that followed. Terman wanted his tests to be administered by a 'trained tester working with one child at a time'. He urged that all children should be tested and since he was disclosing 'innate ability' he 'could sort all children into their proper stations in life' (Gould 1992, p176). However, when Terman embarked on the ambitious project of testing all children in American schools, tests were reduced to 5, and testing required 30 minutes to complete. Terman believed that he could identify innate intelligence in this way and predicted that 'in the near future ... high grade defectives' will be subject to 'the surveillance and protection of society', and this would curtail 'the reproduction of feeble-mindedness ... and the elimination of crime, pauperism, and industrial inefficiency' (Terman 1919, p6 & p7).

Terman continued to interpret test results on the assumption that the IQ scores he obtained were indicative of an inherited capacity, and that the environment played no part in the measures achieved. Like others committed to eugenics, and the social arrangements that favoured capitalism, he often used dubious methodologies to promote his assertions, which enabled him to identify those responsible for societies' ills. For instance, he tested hoboes and the unemployed but supressed the total results and focussed on the low 25%. During the depression years Terman shifted in his views, and in 1937, he acknowledged that children from the 'lower economic strata' were able to show a rise in IQ after school attendance and he proposed that further research on environmental influence should be undertaken (Terman and Maud 1937).

The American government, convinced by the propaganda of Goddard and Terman, employed the psychologist Yerkes, R. M. to test 1.75 million army recruits during World War I. He worked with Goddard and Terman, and they used three test procedures. Literate recruits would be given the Army Alpha, a written examination, and recruits who could not complete the Alpha were to be given a visual test, the Army Beta. Subjects who failed in the Beta would be recalled and given an individual examination using Binet's scales. Recruits were then graded from A to E with plus and minuses. These results were then intended to be used in determining military placement.

The tests delivered to large groups were culturally loaded and 'strictly timed'. Although some explanation was given to those recruits taking the Alpha none was given to the Beta recruits. 'Procedures varied so much from camp to camp that results could scarcely be collated and compared' Gould tells us (op cit p201). A tester complains

> the room in which the examination is held is filled too full of men. As a result, the men who are sitting in the rear of the room are unable to hear clearly and thoroughly enough to understand the instructions.
>
> Yerkes (1921, p106)

The allocation of recruits to the Beta form was inconsistent and often illiterate recruits were pushed into the Alpha examination to avoid large Beta groups. This distorted results and corrupted the agreed methodology.

Gould shows that when recruits who scored D on Alpha were given the opportunity to take the Beta, they usually gained a higher grade, and it was clear from the detail provided by Yerkes that the score of black recruits 'improved substantially' (op cit p203). In Yerkes' figures, there were clear indications that subjects who had received more schooling achieved better scores. But Yerkes, perversely argued that 'Failure to attend school ... must reflect a disinclination based on low intelligence' (op cit p219). Yerkes also noticed in relation to 'foreign born recruits' that average test scores rose consistently in relation to the years of residence in the United States, but he was reluctant to admit to any situational or social and environmental element at work in the tests. The results of the Army tests, Gould suggests, 'could have provided an impetus for social reform'. But, as far as the psychologists were concerned measures or numbers could not relate to anything but *inherited* intelligence (Gould op cit p221).

Spearman studied the scores from different mental tests and where he noticed that the correlation coefficients were positive he inferred the presence of 'G' or general intelligence. Gould observes that 'correlations between tests are usually far weaker than correlations between two parts of a growing body' (op cit p251). That is to say, developmentally as legs grow so do arms, so measures will change proportionately, but such a strong relation does not exist between the numbers from different mental tests. Gould argues that correlations, even where strong, do not disclose the presence of an entity that is causal and that there are other ways of simplifying the large sets of data involved which would eliminate the existence of 'G'.

Sir Cyril Burt researching and writing in Britain between 1909 and 1972 studied identical twins 'raised apart' and he undertook studies of close relatives. His early published papers supported the thesis that intelligence could be identified as a 'thing' to be located in the brain, having a 'definite degree of heritability', and that it could be measured as a single number, thus providing a 'ranking of people according to the amount of it they possess' (Gould 1992, p239). However, the numbers in his early papers were faked, and data was shown to be manufactured. This revelation was slow to emerge but it did not, seemingly, affect Sir Cyril's career, who probably invented his co-authors (see Rutherford 2022, footnote, p167).

In the 1940s Burt championed the factor analysis undertaken by Spearman and he argued that correlations were capable of disclosing hereditable causation. Like the Americans, Burt aimed to 'deduce from an empirical set of test measurements a single figure for each single individual' (Burt 1940, p176). He never doubted the existence of inheritable intelligence despite encountering evidence that suggested environment and education impacted the results obtained in his tests. He wrote 'the facts of genetic inequality, ... are something we cannot escape' and 'A definite limit to what children can achieve is inexorably set by the limitations of their innate capacity' (Burt 1959, p28 in Gould op cit p285).

This 'vision of a single ranking', showing an 'inherited ability', was attractive to the British Government and gained political influence via the Butler Education Act of 1944, which produced the 11+ examination, visited on all state schools, and determined the future higher educational opportunities for 11 year olds. Eleven years of age was regarded as the age at which 'G' stabilised. Burt argued that he was providing the opportunity for 'disadvantaged children' but he did not believe that 'many people of high intelligence lay hidden in the lower classes' (Gould 1992, p295).

L. L. Thurstone professor of psychology at the University of Chicago published his research papers between 1924 and 1955, he used factor analysis to 'discover the mental faculties' which he referred to as 'Vectors of the Mind' (Thurstone 1935, p53). He argued that 'G' was only an average which would change according to the number and nature of tests that were put together. By re-arranging the statistical results of tests into vectors, Thurston was able to argue that tests measure a number of independent 'primary mental abilities' (PMAs) (Gould 1992, p301). He identified seven PMAs, verbal comprehension, word fluency, number, spatial visualisation, associative memory, perceptual speed, and reasoning, and he believed that children should not be judged by a single 'number' (op cit p305). Burt and Spearman responded to Thurstone by suggesting that he had simply produced an alternative mathematics for the same data that showed the existence of 'G'. Both approaches, Gould reminds us, are 'plagued with the conceptual error of reification' (p310), positive correlations between test results, however mathematically arranged, cannot be taken as a clear identification of 'G' or 'PMAs' and neither do they support, by themselves, either an argument for a purely hereditary acquisition of intelligence or a purely environmental acquisition.

But what is intelligence? Gould does not mention Hebb (1949) who argued that there could be two ways of understanding the concept of intelligence. 'Intelligence A' referred to a potential, or innate capacity, that an intact brain, and an intact neural metabolism, might possess, while 'intelligence B' is exhibited through the functioning of the brain and neural metabolism, at any given moment. 'Intelligence A' is essentially an abstraction, a hypothesis, a potential, assumed to exist. The assumption, or hypothesis, in relation to 'intelligence B' is that the test and the test situation are capable of disclosing the functioning of the brain of a given subject in such a way that a number can be assigned to it. What we know is that intelligence tests are designed to provoke particular behaviours, and for the individual to gain any score a behaviour, assessed as being intelligent, must be recorded by the examiner. This does leave open a number of questions, for instance, what behaviours exhibit intelligence, and why such behaviours might not appear in an individual's repertoire, at any given moment.

Gould does give us some description of the early tests, their cultural and educational content, and some good description of the contexts in which tests were administered, for example in the army tests and in the testing of immigrants. His particular interest is in the statistical analysis that psychologists have used to support their claims. He argues that despite the 'elaborate statistical work performed by testers during the last 50 years', there has been 'no independent confirmation that the tests measure intelligence' (Gould 1992, p175 & p177).

Currently, the favoured test for children is the Wechscler Intelligence Scale V 2014, the tests are designed to measure a range of different abilities, including verbal comprehension, and visual and spatial reasoning. There is some measure of process speed and tests include picture sorting, arithmetic and memory. Psychologists, today, are more focussed on testing in the spirit of Binet (Binet and Simon 1939), to gain a clearer picture of a child's mental processing over a range of tests and subtests so as to be able to suggest remedial measures in learning situations.

We do need to be aware that the idea that inheritance is *the* determinate factor in relation to intelligence, still exerts considerable influence. Jensen in 1979 using the same arguments as Spearman to propose the existence of 'G' was arguing for a difference between populations, claiming that there was an 'innate deficiency of intelligence amongst blacks' (Gould op cit p319). Stephen Hsu, in the Guardian newspaper 25 May 2019 P13, is described as 'a leading US scientist', he has a company called Genomic Prediction. He suggests it will be possible to predict IQ in an embryo, within 'if not the next five years, the next 10 certainly'; and Professor Simon Fishel, in the same article asks, 'what's wrong with ranking an embryo if you can rank a child?' The desire to assess individuals in utero, before birth, is usually linked to the wish to avoid abnormalities, disease and trauma at birth. The problem, for me, with Professor Fishel's approach, is the link to IQ. Were it to become possible to assess or predict the future IQ of an unborn child, it would serve as the continuation of a particular political agenda, a political desire to rank individuals at birth and assign value, to determine social destiny.

Intelligence testing is important in another way, it gives support to the Medical Sciences in confirmation of impairment, often where no clear indication of neurological damage or disease is present from clinical investigations, but where perhaps there is some 'malform', and suggestion of developmental delay from behaviour. Developmental, and or Cognitive, Psychologists in their turn seek support from the Medical sciences in confirming their findings in relation to behaviour and development, as we have seen above, and testing itself requires some support from Developmental Psychologists in the development of tests. Much of testing is dependent on statistics, but as the history that Gould supplies shows, the statistics in themselves do not confirm the existence of an heredity substance, capacity, or potential, we call 'intelligence', although tests may confirm that an individual can complete a range of identified mental operations, in particular situations.

The three discursive domains present in diagnostic assessments are linked. They support each other and adopt a version of mind which gives emphasis to neurological inheritance and neurological activity, where abstraction, mental representations, and hypothecating characterise mental activity. Principally it is almost all done in the head.

The Location of Mind

We all feel we know what intelligence is when we see it, because we have received, and developed, ideas of what constitutes intelligent behaviour, in relation to age and situation. In our everyday talk in relation to the mind, which must be present if we were to witness intelligent behaviour, we are often preoccupied with 'the thing in the head' as Ryle (1973 (1949), p40) puts it. However, spatial metaphors are often in use when it comes to the mind, things can be held in the mind, and we can be out of our mind, our minds can be elsewhere. But where should we look for the mind, if not in the head, which is where it is located in the discourses we have been examining? Perhaps the 'numskulls' can help us (Figure 1).

As we can see, at the top of the strip, the Numskulls are presented as living and working in Edd's head. Brainy is at the top left, he is the first homunculus [a little man (sic)], the personification of a faculty, an agent that performs a function), that we encounter. Brainy is first in many senses, as a leader and initiator of activity, and as the strip shows he has to make sense of written messages that reach him from a machine in the corner of the Brain Dept. We might ask where do the messages come from? One thing to note is that the messages are often puzzling for Brainy.

The Brain Dept is just behind the Eye Dept where Blinky works, below them on another level is Radar who responds to the sounds that reach him via Edd's ears, in front of him is Snitch who is responsive to smells, and relaxing on Edd's tongue in the lower floor, is Cruncher who is in charge of the mouth department, which has access to Edd's stomach. Brainy interacts with Blinky, Radar, Snitch and Cruncher,

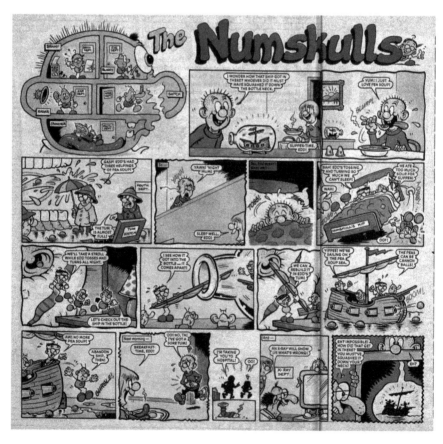

Figure 1 The Numskulls. From the Beano (1999). Used by kind permission of DC Thomson & Co Ltd.

and this, maybe, exemplifies Brainy's access to sensory information and his link to other, more distant bodily regions – for instance, the stomach which Cruncher ensures is filled with food.

Following on from the cross section of Edd's head the first two frames of the strip appear. We are introduced to Edd and his mother. Edd's attention is captured by the ship in the bottle, an object that exudes a magical aura. Edd is astonished and his mind is filled with wonder. How did that ship get in the bottle? This question could explain Brainy's puzzling message at the start of the whole strip. The question remains central to the story, but first, there is his mother's food, Edd's favourite pea-soup. He slurps down his soup while his eyes are fixated on the ship in the bottle.

In frame three we learn that Edd has had three helpings of Pea-soup and this keeps Cruncher, and what looks like Brainy and Blinky, suitably dressed, busy. So next with a full stomach, Edd retires to bed under the watchful eye of his indulgent mother. Notice the fly that seems to have passed through Edd's head. Now his mind is elsewhere, he is falling asleep, and the fly implies that Edd has nothing between his ears at this moment in time. If the mind is usually found within the head, and the mind and brain are one, then an absent mind implies an absent brain, or it could be that Edd has an impairment of some sort that allows the fly a free passage through or past his brain.

In frames 5 and 6 we witness the result of Edd's excess? As sleep is not possible Brainy and his friends, who personify the sensory element, are disturbed and become active in the night. They exit Edd's head via his ear. We could see this as Edd dreaming about the ship, dreaming of the solution to the problem that has occupied him in the day, because of the disturbance in his stomach. We are told by Freud that the dream is shaped by the pre-conscious which wants to maintain sleep [Freud 1983 (1900)]. Maybe frames 6–11 show us the dream as it appears to consciousness, after secondary revision.

This interpretation, that the problem is solved by Brainy alone while residing in Ed's head, would support the natural intellectualist view of the mind. The intellectualist view of the mind, presents mind as being firmly located within the head of the thinker, and to 'engage in action one must' ... first ... 'contemplate some proposition' (Radman 2013, p369 & p370). Every action is preceded by a plan, and we must all be planners who are aware of our 'moves' beforehand. It is intelligent planning, or propositional thought, that results in intelligent performances according to the intellectualist view.

But we are also given another possibility that it is not a dream of Edd's at all, but the disturbed faculties (the little men) are *really* engaging with the bottle and its contents in a direct and physical way, which is precisely what material reality demands. 'I see how it got into the bottle it comes apart!' exclaims Brainy as he now begins to use his *hands*. Contemplation and dream production are not enough to solve the problem that excites Edd's wonder, neither is Brainy's planning, if he made a plan, instead it is his hands that enables him to discover the secret of the ship and the bottle.

When the little men 'check out' the ship in the bottle we could say that an analysis takes place in frames 8 and 9, but it is not the decoding of messages, or an engagement with representations and symbolic material, that solves the problem, but instead it is the manual which brings the material world into a relationship with all the bodily faculties (Brainy, Blinky, Snitch, Radar and Cruncher), which produces an appreciation of how the ship got into the bottle. We could suggest, that there should be another little man, or little woman, a homunculus, in Edd's head with very large hands, to illustrate the importance of hands to Brainy, Blinky, Snitch, Radar and Cruncher, except it might be difficult to know where to locate her or him.

Hands, when engaged in an interaction with the material element, are capable of gaining a particular understanding of objects properties and possibilities. Brainy and his friends are thus tempted to play with the ship from the bottle, in Edd's 'tum' – frames 8, 9, 10 and 11. They play until the soup runs out and then return to where they are usually found, in Edd's head.

But there is no fun for Edd, as we see, he feels sore in the morning and cannot eat the sausage and eggs his mother prepares for him. In the last two frames, Edd is in the hospital as his mother takes him there. He is x-rayed. The professorial doctor is confident that he can diagnose the problem but in the final frame the doctor is left with the same problem that preoccupied Edd; 'How did that get in there?' The doctor's astonishment is different from Edd's wonder. The doctor feels he is a witness to the 'impossible'. We the readers know that, of course, it entered Edd's stomach via his ear! Perhaps the really significant frame in the whole strip is number 13, which is not quite a frame because it doesn't have a border, it is the picture of Edd's smelly sock, with Edd and his mother in the distance. This contingent element tells us that the strip is, after all, a comedy that I should never have treated to such a serious descriptive interpretation.

While the strip emphasises on the importance of the brain, and its relation to the body, especially in its sensory aspect, it also illustrates that thinking takes place in a cultural and social context, in Edd's home, and it requires some engagement with the material world. This is where the mind makes its appearance, when the body and the hands are involved.

This is the counter argument to the intellectualist view, as Ryle puts it:

The clown's trippings and tumblings are the workings of his mind … but the similar trippings and tumblings of a clumsy man are not the workings that man's mind. For he does not trip on purpose. Tripping on purpose is both a bodily and a mental process, but it is not two processes, … [there is no] … counterpart performance to that which is taking place … [no] … cogitative shadow-operation which we do not witness.

Ryle (1973 (1949), p34)

Radman (2013) argues, 'What conscious perception tells the agent may prove not to be relevant' (p375) and the hand has its own intelligence. Further, it is our use of objects and our experience of them that is critical in developing our awareness of intentionality, which often comes later. The mind then is more than information processing that takes place in the brain.

Clark (2013) points out that Ryle [1973 (1949)] and Dennett (1991) both consider the concept of mind as more akin to 'timekeeping than like the concept of a thing that keeps time (e.g. a watch)'. 'Timekeeping does not have parts … Brains have parts. Bodies have parts' and 'bodies, contribute often in subtle and unexpected ways, to the skills and capacities we identify as mental and as cognitive' (Clark 2013, p265).

Roesch (2013), who researches the theoretical foundations for Robotics, suggests that mind is the body and the hand in a continuous unfolding of interacting 'enactions' … 'embedded in the environment' (p412). Geertz (1993), from anthropology, argues that 'thinking is primarily an overt act conducted in terms of the objective materials of the common culture' and mental processes are situated, they have their place 'at the scholars desk or the football field, in the studio or lorry driver's seat … ' (p83), and Bruner (1990), from the perspective of cognitive psychology, asserts that '*logos* and *praxis* are culturally inseparable' (p81). It is in the world, where the hands are in use, where we should be looking for mind, for the mental processes, or the thinking that shapes our becoming selves. 'In the head', 'can and should be always dispensed with' says Ryle [1973 (1949), p40]. But this might be a difficult habit to extinguish.

References

Archard, D. 1993. *Children: Rights and Childhood.* Routledge, London.

Beano 1999. *The Numskulls.* DC Thomson & Co Ltd., Dundee.

Binet, A. & Simon, T. 1939 (1911). *A Method of Measuring the Development of the Intelligence of Young Children.* Courier Company, Lincoln.

Bradley, B. S. 1991. Infancy as Paradise, *Human Development* 34: 35–54.

Bruner, J. 1990. *Acts of Meaning.* Havard University Press, Cambridge, London.

Bruner, J. & Feldman, C. 1993. Theories of Mind and the Problem of Autism. Chap. 13. In: Baron-Cohen, S., Tager Flusberg, H. & Cohen, D. J. (Eds.) *Understanding Other Minds – Perspectives from Autism.* Oxford University Press, Oxford, New York, Tokyo, pp. 267–291.

Burman, E. 2017. *Deconstructing Developmental Psychology – 3rd Edition.* Routledge, Abingdon, Oxon, New York.

Burt, C. 1940. *The Factors of the Mind.* University of London Press, London.

Burt, C. 1959. The Examination at Eleven Plus, *British Journal of Educational Studies* 7: 99–117.

Chen, H. 2017. *Atlas of Genetics Diagnosis and Counselling – 3rd Edition.* Springer, New York.

Clark, A. 2013. Gesture as Thought? In: Radman, Z. (Ed.) *The Hand, an Organ of the Mind – What the Manual Tells the Mental.* The MIT Press, Cambridge, London.

Dennett, D. 1991. *Consciousness Explained.* Little, Brown, Boston.

Fan, Y. T., Decety, J., Yang, C. Y., Liu, J. L. & Cheng, Y. 2010. Unbroken Mirror Neurons in Autism Spectrum Disorders, *Journal of Child Psychology and Psychiatry* 51(9): 981–988.

Fonagy, P. 2001. *Attachment and Psychoanalysis.* The Other Press, New York.

Fonagy, P. 2003a. The Interpersonal Interpretative Mechanism. In: Green, V. (Ed.) *Emotional Development in Psychoanalysis, Attachment Theory and Neuroscience: Creating Connections.* Brunner-Routledge, London, pp. 107–128.

Fonagy, P. 2003b. *Attachment to Ideas: The Status of Attachment Theory in Psychoanalytical Thought.* Unpublished Paper to Centre for the Advancement of Psychoanalytical Studies.

Foucault, M. 2000. The Abnormals. pp 51–57 In: Rabinow, P. (Ed.) and Hurley, R. et al. (Trans.) *Ethics Subjectivity and Truth – Essential Works of Foucault 1954–1984.* Penguin Books, London, New York, Victoria Australia, Ontario Canada, New Delhi, Albany New Zealand, Rosebank South Africa.

Foucault, M. 2003. *The Birth of the Clinic.* Sheridan, A. M. (Trans.). Routledge Classics, Routledge, London, New York.

Freud, S. 1983 (1900). *The Interpretation of Dreams.* The Pelican Freud Library, Penguin Books, Middlesex.

Gallese, V. & Goldman, A. 1998. Mirror Neurons and the Simulation Theory of Mind-Reading, *Trends in Cognitive Science* 2: 493–501.

Geertz, C. 1993. *The Interpretation of Cultures.* Fontana Press, London.

Goddard, H. H. 1914. *Feeble-Mindedness: Its Causes and Consequences.* MacMillan, New York.

Goddard, H. H. 1919. *Psychology of the Normal and Subnormal.* Dodd, Mead and Company, New York.

Goddard, H. H. 1928. Feeblemindedness: A Question of Definition, *Journal of Psycho-Asthenics* 33: 219–227.

Gould, S. J. 1992. *The Mismeasure of Man.* Penguin Books. London, New York, Victoria, Toronto, and Auckland.

Hebb, D. D. 1949. *Organisation of Behaviour.* John Wiley, New York.

Henley, D. 2012. Knowing the Unknowable: A Multidisciplinary Approach to Postmodern Assessment in Child Art Therapy. In: Gilroy, A., Tipple, R. & Brown, C. (Eds.) *Assessment in Art Therapy.* Routledge, Taylor & Francis Group, London, New York.

Hobson, R. P. 1993. Understanding Persons: The Role of Affect. In: Baron-Cohen, S., Tager-Flusberg, H. & Cohen, D. J. (Eds.) *Understanding Other Minds – Perspectives from Autism.* Oxford University Press, New York, Tokyo.

Jenks, C. 1996. *Childhood.* Routledge, London, New York.

Mental Deficiency Act. 1913. Education in England – 2 Nov 2019, available at: http://www.educationengland.org.uk.

Nelson, K., Henseler, S. & Plesa, D. 2000. Entering a Community of Minds: Theory of Mind from a Feminist Standpoint. In: Miller, P. & Scholnick, E. (Eds.) *Towards a Feminist Developmental Psychology.* Routledge, London, New York.

O'Connor, C. & Joffe, H. 2013. How Has Neuroscience Affected Lay Understanding of Personhood? A Review of the Evidence, *Public Understanding of Science* 22(3): 254–268.

Piaget, J. 1972. *Psychology and Epistomology.* Wells, P. (Trans.). Penguin Press. London.

Pintner, R. 1933. The Feebleminded Child. In: Murchison, C. (Ed.) *A Handbook of Child Psychology.* Clark University Press, Worcester.

Radman, Z. 2013. On Displacement of Agency: The Mind Handmade. In: Radman, Z. (Ed.) *The Hand, an Organ of the Mind – What the Manual Tells the Mental.* The MIT Press, Cambridge, London.

Roesch, E. B. 2013. A Critical Review of Classical Computational Approaches to Cognitive Robotics: Case Study for Theories of Cognition? In: Radman, Z. (Ed.) *The Hand, an Organ of the Mind – What the Manual Tells the Mental.* The MIT Press, Cambridge, London.

Rutherford, A. 2022. *Control – The Dark History and Troubling Present of Eugenics.* Weidenfeld & Nicolson, London.

Ryle, G. 1973 (1949). *The Concept of Mind.* Penguin Books, Middlesex.

Suttie, I. D. 1988 (1935). *The Origins of Love and Hate.* Free Association Books, London.

Terman, L. M. 1919. *The Intelligence of School Children.* Houghton Mifflin, Boston.

Terman, L.M. and Merill, Maud A. 1937. *Measuring Intelligence.* A Guide to the Administration of the new revised Stanford-Binet tests of Intelligence. Boston: Houghton MIfflin.

Tredgold, A. F. 1908. *Mental Deficiency (Amentia).* Bailliere, Tindall & Cox, Covent Garden, London. Digitized by the Internet Archive in 2016. https://archive.org/details/b28047667 – accessed 08.08.22.

Trevarthen, C., Aitken, K., Papoudi, D. & Roberts, J. 1996. *Children with Autism: Diagnosis and Interventions to Meet Their Needs – 2nd Edition.* Jessica Kingsley Publishers, London, Philadelphia.

Yerkes, R. M. 1921. Psychological Examining in the United States Army. In *Memoires of the National Academy of Sciences*, Volume 15. National Academy of Sciences, Washington D.C., 890 pp.

Chapter 2

Case Studies

Case studies, the reading of and the writing of, have been central to my Art Therapy practice. They have entertained, inspired and perplexed, and in training generated anxiety, but more importantly, they have prompted me to access theory and to seek an understanding through research. If case study is a problematic research methodology, it has, nevertheless, been essential to the growth of Art Therapy, and It is hard to imagine Art Therapy without this form of writing and research, just as it would be difficult to imagine Psychoanalytic and Analytical therapies, Client Centred, Existential, Humanistic, Cognitive, and Play therapies, without the support of case studies to argue for theoretical constructs and forms of practice.

Case Studies as Research

Whether they concern themselves with contemporary or past practices, case studies are necessarily confined to time and place, and specificity is a characteristic but not an objection to treating case studies as research. Individual case studies ($N=1$ as Gilroy (2011) ironically characterises it) can 'can show what is possible' but not necessarily 'what is common' (Galatzer-Levy et al. 2000, p238). They do not just provide answers that conform to a priori assumptions and paradigms, but through their particularity, they enable fresh schemas to be constructed which can be assessed in relation to other individual cases. According to Yin (1989), case studies are 'generalizable to theoretical propositions'. Yin is writing from a sociological perspective, and his comments support McLeod's (2010) argument, constructed from a psychotherapeutic perspective, which asserts that case studies are good vehicles for developing theory.

All treatments, or cases, in Art Therapy or Art Psychotherapy can be characterised as 'research' in so far as each case, client, child or service user, or member(s) of a group, each therapist, and each meeting, raises questions and problems, which require some application of theory and method to enable that necessary, continuous assessment of practice. Problems have their origins; they may relate to the context in which the work is situated, to the resistance of the therapist, or to the patient's difficulty in engaging in the work, perhaps in responding to the demand – 'make use of the art materials', or in the demand for communication. Whatever the

DOI: 10.4324/9781003360056-3

difficulties or the nature of the obstacles faced by the therapist, they are likely to be numerous and she is likely to need to find ways of researching her experience. Much of this problem-solving will take place in clinical supervision and this may be the arena where research is seen as opportune or necessary in relation to the case. Importantly, case studies can also provide an occasion for a collaborative engagement with clients in research. See Dalley et al. (1993) for a helpful exploration of three critical viewpoints, the client, the therapist, and the clinical supervisor.

Case studies can provide a 'supporting role' in meeting the NHS requirement for Evidenced Based Practices (EPB) but as Gilroy (2006, 2011) in her studies of Art Therapy researches indicates, 'qualitative approaches' to research 'have been significantly undervalued' in EBP (Gilroy 2006, p85). Statistical presentations that present outcome measures are seen as having more value than researches whose result is just text, and if the text contains an element of subjective reflection, and foregrounds the use of visual material, it might well be ignored, especially where the interested parties' only consideration is funding. Gilroy responds to this by arguing that where there is 'detail given in relation to the research and its context' and 'transparency' in terms of the researchers 'personal engagement and heuristic process' then 'integrity and credibility' can be established (Gilroy 2006, p85; McLeod 2001).

Text and images appear in the researches of other disciplines, which make use of case studies, for example in anthropology, ethnography, sociology and art history. Gilroy suggests that art therapists, in researching cases, should make full use of visual material and develop visual methodologies, and while there is no 'correct' methodology in relation to case studies, artworks demand a self-aware interpretative frame and process (Gilroy 2011, p9).

Schaverien (1992) provided the profession in Britain with a longitudinal case study that focussed on imagery and the processes related to art production. This research has been foundational in relation to Art Therapy practice in Britain, and in 1995, Schaverien wrote about her research journey. Schaverien's interest was in the 'aesthetic effects', the power to be affected, by 'the picture within the therapeutic relationship'. The method 'was developed as needed', but 'thinking hard' and philosophy were important in this. The patient's works are approached through the 'retrospective review', which looks carefully at all the pictures arranged in a dated sequence. Fresh observations are made and fresh understandings are reached. 'The countertransference is reawakened', Schaverien argues, and in this 'looking back at a process' the therapeutic encounter is disclosed (Schaverien 1995, p30 & p33).

What Schaverien is proposing is that we can think of the writing and the encounter with the art products produced in Art Therapy, as a recovery of a subjectivity, a subjectivity which enables the researcher to approach the 'amorphous area characterised by the often intimate relating of two people and a picture' (Schaverien, 1995 p21).

Edwards stresses that case research is a writing process and a looking that requires thinking, that is critical in relation to 'what we do and why we do it', Edwards (1999). He argues that we cannot 'dispense' with our subjectivity, since 'what we do' [as art therapists] 'belongs to the intermediate area of experience between what is 'real' and what is imagined' – here Edwards refers to Winnicott (1980). He commends case studies that can pay 'serious attention to the individuality of the client'; engage 'with the ... messiness and complexity' of 'process and lived experience'; facilitate the re-examination of 'existing theories; and are inclusive in respect of the 'voice' of the client and therapist (Edwards 1999, p4 & p6).

Case Studies are about telling stories, which is a 'ubiquitous yet fundamental human activity'. If stories 'structure what we believe to be true' and 'false' (Edwards 1999, p7) then there arises the problem that 'Truth and fiction exist on a continuum, and no messages arrive un-coded, innocent of beliefs or persuasion' (Knights 1995, p69 – quoted in Edwards 1999, p7).

Edwards (1999, p5) argues that we are positioned by the 'power relations that sustain' our discursive environment, and he called for the use of a 'critical subjectivity' from art therapists researching cases, and this should involve us in an analysis of the ways in which Art Therapeutic discourses themselves produce subjects, through the reproduction of power relations. Linnell (2010) investigates this issue. 'The individual' is the 'The place where thought gets stuck', she argues. Attention to the discursive rather than the 'intrapsychic' is required. This involves a de-centring of the rational autonomous (modern) subject in our Art Therapy narratives. This is a 'difficult project' but we have to avoid 'expressive' therapies that 're-stage the pathologisation and isolation of the subject, and re-instate the therapist as expert', an expert who re-enforces 'the separation and mystification of the aesthetic sphere' (Linnell 2010, p25). In the development of her thinking Linnell reaches an understanding that doubt is, itself, a necessary ethical resource, and this surely has to be present in all forms of case study.

In my introduction, I presented an ontological claim. Subjects, I proposed, existed bodily as persons and were referred to or represented in practices. My claim draws support from Hegel, in the Phenomenology of Spirit, who presents the subject as a 'bearer of psychological states and processes, the human subject ...' as a 'performer of actions and activities' – see Inwood (1992, p280 & p283). This implies a rational autonomous subject, perhaps, but Butler (2012) stresses that, 'the Hegelian subject is not a self-identical subject who travels smugly from one ontological place to another; it *is* its travels, and *is* every place in which finds itself' (p8, author's emphasis). This is how I prefer to think of the subject. Subjects are situated and on the move, subjectivity then becomes shorthand for that experience of being a particular subject for others, and identity and agency are shared and difficult to apprehend. But how should we think of inter-subjectivity?

In psychoanalysis, the investigation of the notion of *inter*subjectivity has been instigated by Winnicott [1987 (1951)] in his emphasis on 'transitional' phenomena, more recently by Muller (1996) who explores the semiotics of dyadic relations, and by Benjamin (2004), through a focus on recognition and mutuality. Intersubjectivity is there from the beginning, and the dyadic relation has a relation to a third Other. Other with a capital 'O' for Lacan is language, speech and law, the symbolism which arrives from another place (see Evans 1996), but I would also want to use the large 'O' to reference the many others that constitute a world, and I want to include the material practices and the social exchanges that particular settings generate, in this third. This thinking about subjects and places, or settings, will be enlarged, I hope, as the book proceeds but first I wish to give an account of researches that shows how the beginnings of this way of thinking emerged for me.

Some Personal Researches

What follows is an account of some case study researches which I undertook in 1992 and 2011 (see Tipple 1992, 2011). The research journeys I present are intended to demonstrate that a clarification in relations to fundamentals is possible, through a reflective and 'critical subjectivity', and that this clarification enables further questions to be applied to the practice of Art Therapy, in relation to subjects and subjectivity.

Alfred

My first serious attempt at researching a case, after my initial training, focussed on a young man with a severe learning disability, aged 22, whom I have called 'Alfred'. He had been in long-term care since the age of 7. Alfred had no speech, and his communicative resources seemed limited, and in the hospital notes, a diagnosis of 'Childhood Psychosis' was recorded.

Alfred's preference was to paint A2 sheets in one uniform colour, paying particular attention to the removal of brush marks to gain a flat uniform surface of unmodulated colour. Two immediate questions arose, should I intervene in his processes to increase communication, and what could painting, in my attentive presence, mean to him … and his therapist?

Answering these questions lead me to explore researches that lead away from the object relations approach that had, in this early part of my career, begun to inform my thinking. Dubowski (1985) and Rees (1995) had undertaken some researches which explored the work of the more severely learning disabled residents living in large hospitals, using ethology to develop a methodology. Ethology is the science of animal behaviour, but there were ethologists who wanted to apply their science to the human situation, for example Polsky and Chance (1979) who had researched the use of physical space in long-stay psychiatric hospitals.

Dubowski was interested in comparing the mark-making of normal children, at the pre-representational phase to the mark-making of his clients. He concluded that his clients were less experimental than young children, and he described the work of his four subjects, as lacking in initiative. He reported that little attention was given to the marks, and his subjects sought 'comfort' when marking. Importantly, Dubowski did establish the idea, in my mind at least, that manipulating the mark-making conditions, as he did, by, for example, providing marked paper to his subjects, might be a way of communicating via the material in use, and might encourage initiative and the development of relationship.

Rees (1995) observed her patients on the ward and in the Art Therapy sessions. She was interested in the use of the physical space of the ward and the use of the space offered by the paper when painting. She was able to show a link between her observations on the ward and the painting which was often concerned with a reinforcement of boundaries. For instance, on the ward, a young man who spits on his hands and sweeps them along the floor, and reaches for the corners and the edge of the room, when painting, in the Art Therapy setting, pays attention to the edges and corners of the paper. Rees argued that an emotional need was at work here, and the use of a spatial intelligence enables the individual to find a more secure sense of self in the setting.

The coloured sheets that Alfred produced reminded me of Ad Reinhardt who was associated with the Abstract Expressionists, he writes: 'no illusions, no representations, no associations ... no paint qualities, no impasto, no experiments ... no nonsense ... no confusing painting with everything that is not painting' (Reinhardt 1965 (1952), p132 & p133). Reinhardt was emptying his work of referential content and reaching for the incontrovertible bedrock in painting, and Alfred, it seemed to me, understood what was required when presented with brushes and paints and sheets of paper, and his choice, his personal brief, was to adhere to the fundamentals of the task as signified in the material element supplied by the therapist.

So, thinking of what I learnt from Dubowski, I did offer Alfred a paper sheet on which I had painted, in his presence, a circle outlined in orange. He filled the circle in orange allowing a little colour to just go beyond the outline. When given a green outline, he filled it in green. Alfred appeared to enjoy this sort of game, sometimes with three different coloured circles to respond to on one sheet. I then began painting on some separate paper in the sessions, while he painted. The essential differences in my paintings were that they were divided into *two* contrasting colours – perhaps I was telling Alfred that there were two of us here together, painting. Alfred laughed when he saw me paint and tapped his chin (a positive or affirmative sign). However, he was not immediately influenced by my painting and preferred to paint using one colour. As Alfred worked through the colours in the pallet one by one, and because he used paint liberally, his pots of colour soon became empty. It was then necessary to move on to a fresh pot and a fresh colour. This process in time, led him to relax in his desire for an homogenous finish in his painting and he began to accept contrasts resulting from the changes in colour. He surprised me on occasions, showing evidence of a change of mind, breaking his characteristic rhythmic movements, he stopped, and removed paint from his brush, scraping it on the side of a pot carefully, he then moved to a fresh, more deliberately chosen, sometimes contrasting, colour.

In my retrospective viewing of Alfred's work, I noticed that, as our relationship became more established through routine, movement and gesture began to play a larger part in his painting. His activity was affected by what was happening to him at a bodily level, and by events around him, in his immediate environment, for instance, when we were working in the dining room of the ward, he noticed that, in the dayroom seen through the glass partition, sandwiches were being handed out. I allowed him to fetch some sandwiches, and after the enjoyment of the sandwich, the subsequent rhythm, and energy in the gesture of his painting, reflected his happy mood. Bodily movement I recognised then, betrays or expresses emotion, and this emotional movement can be communicated through the movement of paintbrush or marker – there is an indexical sign here (Peirce 1985). The movement visible in the paint surface refers to the movement of the hand, arm and body, through our appreciation of the causal and contiguous relationship.

It has been suggested that facial expressions sensed by the individual as she or he makes them help that individual determine their own emotional state (Tomkins 1962–1963). The English philosopher Midgley (1979) has commented on this aspect of communication:

> throwing something down on learning a piece of news does the same clarifying job, both for the thrower and for others, as swearing. It manifests his feelings not just as an undifferentiated flood, but as a certain kind and degree of annoyance, indignation, despair or whatever. In such ways do we make ourselves understood both to ourselves and each other.
>
> (p246)

Midgley brings the body and the intersubjective perspective into view in relation to the expression of emotions, and I began to see that I had some impact on the direction of Alfred's work, through my management of the setting, and my engagement in the material element – paint, brushes and paper. In this sense, the painting should be understood as the product of at least two people, of an encounter and an exchange. Nevertheless, the achievement of personal expression, in my presence, with the resources available, was Alfred's.

After this study and writing I could now appreciate that expression takes place in a setting, and it is mediated by a material element, and in Art Therapy it usually entails an exchange between people. A 'setting' implies a space, which is organised to encourage a particular engagement with tools and materials, a particular form of material practice, and relationship with others.

PhD Research

My study of Alfred's painting was published in 1992. The PhD research which I now wish to describe below also appeared in print (see Tipple 2011, 2012).

When working in Hospital B I was also employed in a multi-disciplinary team (MDT) linked to the local Child and Adolescent Mental Health Services, which I called 'Chestnut House'. The team offered consultations to families and children where a question of Paediatric Disability, or Neuro Developmental Disorder, had been raised by the local Paediatricians or local Child and Adolescent Psychiatrists. Personnel included Clinical Psychologists, a Consultant in Paediatric Neurology, sometimes registrars in Child and Adolescent Psychiatry, a Physiotherapist, a Speech and Language Therapist, a Social Worker, a Teacher with Special Needs expertise, a Music Therapist and an art therapist (Myself).

As the art therapist at Chestnut House, my main activity was to participate in the multi-disciplinary assessment process which was aimed at reaching a 'differential diagnosis' in relation to the children referred. The Art Therapy element of this larger (MDT) assessment was usually a single hourly session, which was routinely recorded on video, except in those instances where families, and/or children did not give consent. After the assessment, I was expected to produce a report for the team.

Intimidated by the knowledge and confidence of the other professionals, who seemed to be very clear about how they should assess and how they should interpret the results of their work, I was uncertain. What could I discover in an hour-long assessment using the tools of Art Therapy? My psychodynamic self only rarely found expression in this team work and I was not confident in giving an opinion in relation to diagnosis.

As the team encouraged research I decided to research this Art Therapy Assessment since it seemed to offer me an opportunity to look at the interaction in the setting in detail and to explore the use of materials, by the child and by the therapist, in this unusual situation.

I wanted to know, if through the use of a discourse analysis, I could reach an expanded comprehension of the adult's and the child's relation to art making. Would an analysis of documents, videos and art products provide a richer account of relationships and practices? In engaging with this question I decided to explore the literatures that professionals within the team were not familiar with, and the literatures that I had not made use of in any systematic way in my psychodynamic practices in the hospital, and so I turned to Sociological, Art Historical, Semiotic, Philosophical and cultural literatures.

The research was retrospective and can best be characterised as a heuristic exploration of discourse. I drew upon a flexible definition of discourse, that was 'proposed' by Foucault [2002 (1972)], which would be capable of encompassing written communications and literatures, speech, practices which entails both spatial organisation and the use of tools and materials, ceremonial activity and the sharing of visual products.

I choose to research assessments that had been completed, where I had no further involvement with the child or family, but where parents and children had given permission for me to use material held by the MDT, this included videos, drawings, paintings and clay sculpture, documents from referrers and documents produced by the clinic. I presented four cases in the final PhD. The detail was important to me, and analysing documents and video recordings, creating transcripts and studying Art products took time.

Reading Foucault [2003 (1963), 1972, 1991 (1977), 2002 (1994)] enabled me to examine the documentary material and appreciate assessment as a production of subjects, that is the production of the child with developmental problems. Goffman

[1971 (1959), 2005 (1967)] helped me examine the social interaction in the video material, which encouraged me to notice the theatrical nature of the space and the relation of the protagonists, the referred child and the art therapist (myself), to the setting and the task. From an Art Historical perspective, Baxandall's (1985, 1991) account of intentionality and ekphrasis (a written or verbal description of a visual experience) helped me produce an interpretative description of the art products that were produced; and Austin (1962), with his emphasis on speech acts, Peirce (1985) on semiotics, and Hodge and Kress (1988) on social semiotics, helped me analyse the production and exchange of messages which constituted the texts that were generated in the assessment encounter.

I presented each case (an individual child in assessment) as three 'subjects', according to the research material I was examining. First the documentary subject; the child as represented in the clinical documents by others; the ekphrastic subject; the child as seen through my description of my visual experience of art products, supported by illustrations; and finally the discursive subject; the child as she or he appeared in the transcript produced from the video recording.

The documentary subject takes the form of a story, a narrative that develops around the referred child. The referred subject fits the category of the unusual/not normal compared with his or her peers and there is a disturbance, in the family, and/ or at nursery or school. 'Annie' for instance, is described by her parents as a good baby, one who loves books and retells stories. But it is difficult to gain her attention and her speech is repetitious. 'Damien's' parents produced three and half A4 pages listing his faults, then they apologise for this; 'We know this sounds all so negative but our fears are not vague and unfounded'.

A classificatory system is constructed by the family, the school and the referring professionals, for example; Damien is described as not having a Neuro-Psychiatric Disorder but as suffering from emotional difficulties. Through further assessment Chestnut House attempts to restore family union through an elaboration of the classificatory system, using the specialist knowledge, held within the team. The team then provides a fresh account of the difference and provides a fresh diagnosis using the criteria from diagnostic manuals (ICD 10 or DSM IV at that time). In this way the not-normal is normalised, the un-natural is naturalised, and if parents are happy with the results of the assessment family union can be restored. For instance, Damien was diagnosed as having Asperger's Syndrome which led to a Statement of Special Educational Need, and the parents were pleased with this result.

The documents show that adults are seen to have the power to disclose the emergent rationality of the child (see Jenks 1996). The documentary subject is the subject as she, or he, is constructed by others through discursive practices, it is the outcome of a 'normalizing society' where a 'technology of power centred on life' produces 'normalizing judgements' (Foucault 1991 (1977), p170).

The ekphrastic subject began with the assumption of a rationality present in the artwork that the children and the therapist produced in the assessment. I have, following Baxandall (1985, 1991) assumed that there were reasons why marks were made and placed as they were, that the products look the way that they do because of purposeful actions on the part of the subject child and/or therapist (myself). While I argued that intentionality was evident, in the sense of purpose or aim, through an appraisal of the art object, intentionality is also created retrospectively through the shifting interpretations that the art object is subject to, in the assessment itself, and later during my researches. In this sense, intentionality is never a settled affair. For instance, in relation to 'Henry's' marking with the felt tip pens, I noticed that his marks, through their character and placement, suggested an exploration of the spatial arrangement of the people in the room, himself, his mother, and the therapist. Further, when Henry was making denser patches he held a position away from the base where he sat, and he ventured out towards the therapist – this is seen on the video. The denser marks reflected the pressure Henry was under to interact with the therapist. Henry was testing proximity.

The ekphrastic subject gives us a subject capable of action, actions which arise from an exchange of objects and materials. The art object was capable of providing a particular stimulus for the participants in the assessment, through the display of visual interest, but chiefly through the indexical, iconic and symbolic capacities that it discloses, when joined to other signifying practices and when shared with others.

The discursive subject is necessarily more complex than the ekphrastic and documentary subject, as it originates from an examination of a broader range of dynamic phenomena. It was an attempt to track the variety of movement of bodies and objects, of speech and of response to visual stimuli, as they appear in the video of the assessment. The discursive subject identifies the production of semiotic material in the assessment, its production and exchange, in this way it presents the messages that constitute the assessment text. Subjects construct a definition of the situation and subjects participate in their own formation, but power relations are contested.

When using the blackboard, Annie is willing to present briefly, a less able self, one who struggles with writing, a self-presentation that is unlikely to produce positive feelings for the performer, but which could please the therapist who is tasked with 'making an assessment'. Following this Annie takes charge of cleaning the blackboard which allows her to erase this presentation. Through mime, Annie then presents herself as a teacher directing the children to create a Christmas image. The imaginary situation is maintained by movement, speech, and the production of a drawing of the 'baby Jesus'. Identifying with the teacher role allows her to direct the therapist, undermining his self-presentation as the adult who gives instruction, thus achieving a reversal in the power relation.

When Henry is prompted to respond to figures made with play-doh by the therapist, Henry creates an imaginary situation. In a violent movement, he lifted up his arm and brought it down suddenly to mime destructive attacks or collisions. Henry vocalises; 'Grrrrwater'. He tears the head of the play-doh figure and he stamps his feet. Here he presented himself as a violent powerful figure who ends the play that the therapist had just begun.

The dramaturgy of movement, making and talk, which the video enabled me to examine closely, gave emphasis to the intersubjective nature of the creative and expressive activity that was able to emerge in the assessment. The power relation imposed upon the setting often gave direction to the themes that protagonists (the adult/child dyad) explored. However, mutuality and a solidarity of sorts *was* possible, albeit briefly, in this setting, especially when the therapist was able to modify the more overt demands of the assessment task.

The Client's Voice in Case Studies

Edwards (1999) commended case studies that were inclusive in relation to the voice of the client. But 'Voice' itself is problematic, especially for the person with Learning Disabilities, in the sense that it is difficult for the person with learning disabilities to find that form in which it is best to communicate, in the situation, so that their message might be received and understood – free from the intervention of 'professional' examination and support. Case studies are originated and concluded by the professionals. It is the therapist, who is in a power relation to the client, who has her, or his, own desire, agenda and commitments, who shapes the study. However, one reason for my using discourse analysis in studying the assessment cases was that I was, or at least, I felt that I was, with the help of recording equipment, able to get nearer to the totality of a situation, and access verbal utterances, and observe movement, alongside interactions with materials. But as all communication is situated introducing recording equipment changes the situation, not always for the better, whether it be an interview or a therapeutic encounter, and power relations shape the resulting transcript and analysis. The setting, context, or situation, is productive in relation to expression and the meaning that art production, bodily movement, and verbal language, generate. The client's 'voice', understood as an expression free from external constraint might be more an expression in favour of an abstract freedom, rather than a possible reality.

The Case Studies in Chapters 4 and 5

The two case studies, which are at the centre of this book appear in Chapters 4 and 5, and can best be characterised as longitudinal researches. They were originally submitted for an academic assignment on a masters course in 1995. When first written the case studies were approached through the lens of Art Therapy informed by Kleinian theory. Both these case studies have now been subjected to a later reflection and critical analysis, informed by the researches described above. Taken together these researches have enabled me to attend with greater awareness to the response to context in Art Therapy, and the material practices and exchanges, which characterise the setting. In brief, by making use of later insights and enlarged interpretational frames, I feel that I am now in a better position to grasp the intersubjective element in these earlier Kleinian-informed practices, and explore the relationship of the therapeutic dyad to the larger Other; the world in which the hospital resident and art therapist were immersed.

I do need to add that the literature relating to Art Therapy and Learning Disabilities has produced interesting case material, chiefly in the form of vignettes, but little in the way of longitudinal studies which focus on one case, over time, in depth. This is what I have wanted to see in the literature. Stack's (1998) study of a 44-year-old man, 'Dillon', diagnosed with severe learning disabilities, living in a large hospital comes close. Stack explores some sessions in detail and gives a good account of the frame that she was using to understand the relationship which developed over the two years that 'Dillon' attended Art Therapy with 'Margaret'. Importantly, the study is well illustrated and attention is given to the art-making, and the setting is described and 'Dillon's' experiences and relation to the setting are given proper attention.

An account of Hospital B, which focusses on its history and the changes in discourses and the development of practices in relation to the hospital population, people with learning disabilities now follows in the next chapter. This is preceded by an account of my personal experiences of institutional life.

References

Austin, J. L. 1962. *How to Do Things with Words.* Oxford University Press, Oxford.

Baxandall, M. 1985. *Patterns of Intention – On the Historical Explanation of Pictures.* Yale University Press, New Haven, London.

Baxandall, M. 1991. The Language of Art Criticism. In: Kemal, S. & Gaskell, I. (Eds.) *The Language of Art History.* Cambridge University Press, Cambridge, pp. 67–75.

Benjamin, J. 2004. Beyond Doer and Done To: An Intersubjective View of Thirdness, *Psychoanalytic Quarterly* 73: 5–46.

Butler, J. 2012. *Subjects of Desire – Hegelian Reflections in Twentieth – Century France – With a New Foreword by Phillippe Sabot – Reprint Edition.* Columbia University Press, New York.

Dalley, T., Rifkind, G. & Terry, K. 1993. *The Three Voices of Art Therapy.* Routledge, London.

Dubowski, J. 1985. An Investigation of the Pre-Representational Drawing Activity of Certain Severely Retarded Subjects Within an Institution Using Ethological Techniques, Abstract in Research News, *International Journal of Rehabilitation Research* 8(3): 355. Doctoral Thesis available, Library of Hertforshire College of Art and Design, St Albans Hertfordshire.

Edwards, D. 1999. The Role of the Case Study in Art Therapy Research, *Inscape* 4(1): 2–9.

Evans, D. 1996. *An Introductory Dictionary of Lacanian Psychooanalysis.* Routledge, London and New York.

Foucault, M. 1991 (1977). *Discipline and Punish – The Birth of the Prison.* Sheridan, A. M. (Trans.). Penguin Books, London.

Foucault, M. 2002 (1972). *The Archaeology of Knowledge.* Sheridan Smith, A. M. (Trans.). Routledge Classics, London.

Foucault, M. 2002 (1994). The Subject and Power In: Faubion, J. D. (Ed.) and Hurley, R. et al. (Trans.) *Power – Essential Works of Foucault, 1954–1984*, Volume 3. Penguin Books, London, pp. 326–348.

Foucault, M. 2003 (1963). *The Birth of the Clinic.* Sheridan, A. M. (Trans). Routledge Classics, Routledge, London, New York.

Galatzer-Levy, R., Bachrach, H., Skolnikoff, A. & Waldron, S. 2000. *Does Psychoanalysis Work?* Yale University Press, London.

Gilroy, A. 2006. *Art Therapy, Research and Evidence-Based Practice.* Sage Publications, London, Thousand Oaks, New Delhi.

Gilroy, A. 2011. *Art Therapy Research in Practice.* Peter Lang, Oxford, Bern, Berlin, Bruxelles, Frankfurt am Main, New York, Wien.

Goffman, E. 1971 (1959). *The Presentation of Self in Everyday Life.* Pelican Book, Allen Lane the Penguin Press, Harmondsworth, Middlesex.

Goffman, E. 2005 (1967). *Interaction Ritual – Essays in Face-to-Face Behaviour.* Aldine Transaction, a Division of Transaction Publishers, New Brunswick, London.

Hodge, R. & Kress, G. 1988. *Social Semiotics.* Polity Press, Cambridge.

Inwood, M. 1992. *A Hegel Dictionary.* Blackwell Publishers, Oxford, Cambridge.

Jenks, C. 1996. *Childhood.* Routledge, London, New York.

Knights, B. 1995. *The Listening Reader: Fiction and Poetry for Counsellors and Psychotherapists.* Jessica Kingsley, London.

Linnell, S. 2010. *Art Psychotherapy and Narrative Therapy – An Account of Practitioner Research.* Bentham e Books. University of Melbourne, Australia.

McLeod, J. 2001. *Doing Counselling Research.* Sage, London.

McLeod, J. 2010. *Case Study Research in Counselling and Psychotherapy.* Sage, London.

Midgley, M. 1979. *Beast and Man.* Harvester, Hassocks, Sussex.

Muller, J. P. 1996. *Beyond the Psychoanalytic Dyad – Developmental Semiotics in Freud, Peirce, and Lacan.* Routledge, New York, London.

Peirce, C. 1985. Logic as Semiotic: The Theory of Signs. Reproduced from the Collective Papers of Charles Peirce. In: Innis, R. E. (Ed.) *Semiotics an Introductory Anthology.* Indiana University Press, Bloomington.

Polsky, R. H. & Chance, M. R. A. 1979. An Ethological Perspective on Social Behaviour in Long-Stay Hospitalized Psychiatric Patients, *Journal of Nervous and Mental Disease* 167: 658–667.

Rees, M. 1995. Making Sense of Marking Space – Researching Art Therapy with People Who Have Severe Learning Difficulties. In: Gilroy, A. & Lee, C. (Eds.) *Art and Music Therapy and Research.* Routledge, London, New York.

Reinhardt, A. 1965 (1952). Statement from Contemporary American Painting University of Illonois, Urbana. In: Tuchman, M. (Ed.) *New York School the First Generation: Paintings of the 1940s and 1950s.* New York Graphic Society Ltd., Greenwich.

Schaverien, J. 1992. *The Revealing Image Analytical Art Psychotherapy in Theory and Practice.* Routledge, London.

Schaverien, J. 1995. Researching the Esoteric: Art Therapy Research. In: Gilroy, A. & Lee, C. (Eds.) *Art and Music Therapy Research.* Routledge, London.

Stack, M. 1998. Humpty Dumpty's Shell: Working with Autistic Defence Mechanisms in Art Therapy. In: Rees, M. (Ed.) *Drawing on Difference Art Therapy with People Who Have Learning Difficulties.* Routledge, London, New York.

Tipple, R. 1992. Art Therapy with People Who Have Severe Learning Difficulties. In: Waller, D. & Gilroy, A. (Eds.) *Art Therapy: A Handbook (Psychotherapy Handbooks Series)*. Open University Press.

Tipple, R. 2011. *Looking for a Subject – Art Therapy and Assessment in Autism*. PhD submission, available at Goldsmiths College University, London.

Tipple, R. 2012. The Subjects of Assessment. In: Gilroy, A., Tipple, R. & Brown, C. (Eds.) *Assessment in Art Therapy*. Routledge, Taylor & Francis Group, London, New York.

Tomkins, S. S. 1962–1963. Affect, Imagery, Consciousness. In: Arguile, M. (Ed.) *Bodily Communication*. Methuen, London.

Winnicott, D. W. 1980. *Playing and Reality*. Penguin Books, Harmondsworth.

Winnicott, D. W. 1987 (1951). Transitional Objects and Transitional Phenomena. Chap XVIII. In *Through Paediatrics to Psychoanlalysis – Collected Papers*. Karnac Books Ltd., London, pp. 229–242.

Yin, R. K. 1989. *Case Study Research Design and Methods – Revised Edition*. Applied Social Research Methods Series, Volume 5. Sage Publications, Newbury Park, London, New Delhi.

Chapter 3

Institutions

PART 1

Autobiographical

In an 'austerity Britain', in 1947 when food rationing was in force and the welfare state was in its infancy, I entered the world. My family lived in social housing. The house was situated on a small estate in a Suffolk village. Being near the sea, I liked to listen to the breakers on the shingle shore before falling asleep, and when the dark and wintry North Sea was turbulent and sonorous, I imagined distant places shrouded in mystery. Father was a mystery and shadow. Sometimes a deep sea fisherman, sometimes in small merchant boats travelling up the coast, sometimes working in a factory, he left my mother when I was aged six with seven children to support. I saw little of him but I remember him being drunk, and I remember the smell of him and his bristles when he kissed me goodnight. When Mother tuned into Trawler Band on the big Bush Radio my father's voice calling home was heard. The sound was distant, hidden by a lot of crackle and hiss.

Mother, in her early adolescence, walked across muddy fields to work in the kitchen of a local farmer. Here she learned to cook. This form of employment continued after her marriage, and her skills sustained a large family. There were seven of us, four boys and three girls. I was number six. I acquired a younger brother at 2 years of age. Help was provided by aunties and uncles who lived just three doors away, and the older girls often took care of the younger sibs. Gaining much in the way of sustained attention from Mother was difficult, since she was almost always working. For mother, Sundays were church, and in the evenings, when not resting, it was the Women's Institute.

I experienced deprivation, but there were some good times. When there was money, we could on a Saturday, get fish and chips and pop for lunch. Summer was an exploration of the beach and marshland with other boys from the estate. Often it was a lone wandering in pursuit of some meandering phantasy. My phantasies were fed from imagery shaped by listening to the radio on Saturday mornings, and by the rare Saturday morning visits to the cinema in town, where we watched B movies. Hop-along Cassidy had a big white horse and a big wide white hat. We learned that

DOI: 10.4324/9781003360056-4

he could manage to escape from any perilous situation, tied to the railway by the Indians, that paragon of white supremacy would somehow wriggle free.

Council house children, in the main, were reliant on free school dinners. Wearing my brother's trousers when he outgrew them resulted in the shameful spectacle of appearing in short trousers when all other boys were in long trousers. But, if shame and envy played a part in my early life, relief was felt when Hungarian refugees arrived in the village in 1957, and a more deprived and exotic group was discovered, children without shoes.

Thanks to Sir Cyril Burt and his influence on the Butler Education Act of 1944 (see Chapter 1) I was given the opportunity of failing the 11 plus. In the village Secondary School, where the children were taught no languages, apart from English, and geography was counting the red bits on Mercator's map of the world, I found it difficult to be inspired by the idea of 'education'. It was not until early adolescence, when I 'woke up after Christmas' as one teacher reported, that I began to suspect that I may have missed something that the teachers had been hiding from me.

I did enjoy comics, which were cheap and accessible. My mother, who read herself, encouraged her children by occasionally providing a magazine called 'Look and Learn', which was somewhere between a comic and a 'serious' journal. In this journal, I discovered Van Gogh. As leaving school approached, I began to read books from my Mother's book club. I read Zoo Quest for a Dragon, by David Attenborough – with photos. Attenborough was on show with natives from Borneo, standing close to the cage in which the dragon sulked – how exciting was that?

The need for work was continually stressed at school and at home. We boys must find jobs in the local labour market. Others told me I was 'the best drawer in the school' and when it became near to my leaving the school, it was suggested to me by the deputy head, a good friend of my mother, that I should go to the town's Art School, especially as they seemed keen to recruit me. But my mother was clear that the family could not support this financially, and I had to bring some money in. The idea was dropped. I was only minimally disappointed since the Art Students I had seen in the town with long hair, wore sloppy jumpers and baggy corduroy trousers. They seemed quite alien and I could not imagine myself as part of that club. I was happy to choose a different future.

Through friendship with another boy, I was persuaded to enrol in the local Air Training Corps. Mother approved of the Air Training Corps. I suspected that she liked to see me subjected to military discipline. Certainly, she liked seeing me in uniform. As there was the possibility of some adventure in the Air Training Corps, Summer camps and flying in small aeroplanes and gliders, I was easily convinced that this would be a good thing to do.

Another secret desire was at work here, a desire to leave the village, to get away, to avoid a life of repetitious and monotonous work. To seek adventure – I imagined. So I followed another brother before me who had joined the army to escape, and at 16 years of age I enlisted into the Royal Air Force under the appellation of 'boy entrant'.

As a result, suddenly and catastrophically, I was obliged to move in some other medium, and to relate to some other world. In the first three months, I discovered that verbal abuse could become a natural everyday part of social interaction. We raw recruits, assaulted by insults, were double-marched at speed. We emulated the 'keystone cops' engaged in some mad pursuit, we were rushed from the barracks to the classrooms, to the gym, to the mess, to the parade ground, to the stores, and back again.

On our first visit to the stores we were presented with khaki boiler suits, given boots, coarse woollen socks, and berets to wear. The boots were heavy and made from thick leather, rigid on the bottom and coarsely textured on the uppers. Steel toe and heel plates were driven into the boots. My tender feet suffered badly from blisters. After three months we got our uniforms and we were then taught how to use a brass button stick, how to clean webbing, and how to heat a spoon and remove the texture on our boots, and how to produce the required mirror-like shine through working the polish in circles into the now smooth leather. This was called 'bull'. There were many other tasks which were called 'bull' like this to learn, for example how to polish the linoleum floors in the barrack room, and how to prepare for the daily routine of kit inspections and parades. When we were not required to move our bodies in particular drills, on command, we were subject to inspection. In the classroom, I learned my trade. I was destined for secretarial work and administrative tasks. I learned later that I was being prepared for institutional routine and boredom.

I passed through the training year and Mother was pleased with my new appearance, and I was moved on to my first posting. Soon I was in trouble. Being late back from leave due to a delay on the railways I was greeted with, 'But I told you – there are NO excuses'. Consequentially I was marched before the commanding officer in charge of the secretarial staff and awarded 'seven days restrictions'.

Restrictions, or 'Jankers' as in the common terminology of lowly aircraftmen, entailed extra duties, inspections and the loss of any leisure time. The day began at 5.30 a.m. in the Airmen's Mess serving breakfasts and cleaning up. After an inspection at 6.30 p.m. an evening of 'fatigues' was begun; usually a very unpleasant cleaning task, the more unpleasant the better.

On the evening of the seventh day, I was combatting thick grease in the deep metal sinks of the 'tin room'. Grease was creeping up my arms and I was being pulled into an oily sea on which yellow fatbergs floated. The saturated rags and slippery serving tins became ever more repugnant. I was close to asphyxiation and likely never to reach the end of this episode of 'Jankers', but 9.30 p.m. did arrive to rescue me from my greasy trap. Now I had just 30 minutes to recover and appear in my parade uniform at the guardroom for 10.00 p.m.

It was a tradition, you might say, for the ranks to find ways of quickly responding to this almost impossible timetable, by preparation, having readily available, in the small wardrobe allowed in the barrack room, boots fully polished and wrapped in a duster, white webbing with shining brasses, a clean shirt front, a clean detachable collar – with tie readily attached, and tunic and greatcoat with brass buttons shining. The clean shirt front was just that, no back or sleeves.

I arrived at the Guardroom running; the duty officer, who did not look friendly, was examining his watch. But I was *just* on time, and I was thinking this was my last day of 'Jankers'. The duty officer examined closely the buttons on my greatcoat (it was Winter) and then he studied my shoes – 'Did you polish your boots tonight Airman?' 'Yes Sir I did', I replied. After my response, the duty officer turned to the Sergeant and asked 'Did this airman polish his boots tonight, Sergeant?' As was to be expected, the Sergeant replied, 'No sir, certainly not', without looking at the boots in question. The duty officer repeated his question. Again, I said, 'Yes Sir I did'. Hubris having taken charge, I felt I could not retract, and after all, they were polished as I removed the duster. This resulted in the duty officer asking me to undo my greatcoat so that he could inspect the buttons on my tunic. He found no fault there so he asked me to undo my tunic and he saw the improvised part-shirt. The duty officer, an older warrant officer who clearly knew about these things, was pleased with himself. 'Give this airman another seven days restrictions Sergeant – and make a record of that' he said to the Sergeant, gesturing towards the part-shirt.

In training I quickly learned what it is that is required of the military subject, what forms of instant obedience, what appearances and compliances are expected, and when, and how, one can give an account of oneself. I also learned how this military subject is generated through bodily submissions during drill and in material practices. Once those practices, the raw recruits identified as 'bull', practices that required the skills of polish, appearance and movement had been mastered, then a comfortable repetition became habitual. Such repetitious practices exemplified the 'Disciplinary' power to which I was subject.

Disciplinary power is found in prisons, the military and in large hospitals. It can be regarded as 'a specific technique of a power that regards individuals both as objects and as instruments of its exercise' (Foucault 1991, p170). Discipline inhabits the body and Foucault argues that 'Discipline' 'makes individuals'. But he suggests that there is an obverse to the 'power relationship' established through disciplinary practices. The exercise of this power cannot be divided from 'freedom's refusal to submit' and he uses his own neologism 'agonism' to name a relationship that is 'mutual incitement and struggle; less of a face to face confrontation that paralyzes both sides than a permanent provocation' (Foucault 2002, p342). Freedom is inescapable in the disciplinary situation where power inhabits the body of the subject who is produced and opposes the subjection she, or he, is subject to. However, if power itself produces an opposition, it is also determinate in relation to subjects and subjectivity. If Foucault is right then this feels contradictory, or at best paradoxical. If the individual is determined by disciplinary power, from what source does the individual find the strength and support for the opposition, can it make sense to say from power itself? Butler (1997) takes up this question and argues that it is an iterability, a repetition of the discourses and practices of power, that facilitates a subject's 're-formation', and such a re-formation requires the imaginary.

A repetition allows a spontaneous subject of another sort to emerge. We aircraftmen were all taught how to wear a Beret, the cap badge to the front and the top to be pulled down over to the right side. But everyone made his own, very slight, personal adjustment to this pattern, and, perhaps because this response was universal, it was usually tolerated. Of course, on inspection, it was possible to find that some officer, or non-commissioned officer, did not like your style, and you could then, after some suitable insult had been delivered, be told to re-arrange your headdress. Then the spontaneity of style becomes covert and finds a less readily observable deviation from the norm. It is from these repeated material and bodily practices, often underground, that resistance makes an entrance in the total institution as Goffman (1987) recognises.

This philosophical argument requires that we return to the three people in the situation I described above. The Sergeant was required to endorse the words of the Duty Officer, and the Duty Officer was obliged to represent the authority of the institution, as described in the Station Standing Orders and the manual of Royal Air Force Law. Arriving *just* on time for the final parade and inspection, in the situation described above, was, I now think, the first incitement to combat or 'agonism', and my refusal to agree with the duty officer's estimate in relation to the shoes was a further provocation. I had learned the routine of the disciplinary practices required for the inspection, but in making the practice mine, I had changed the routine in its detail, the most radical element being the part-shirt, in this repetition of the routine where I introduce changes I assert my independence. Really there was no space here for the Aircraftman to speak and offer an opinion, or offer any modifications to the practices that discipline establishes. I was required to be a submissive subject, but something leaks out in the form of opposition, via a repetition, 'the unconscious of power itself', as Butler (1997, p104) puts it. This construction might make sense of Foucault's idea that it is power itself that is productive of resistance.

If opposition in the total institutional setting is unavoidable, in surviving imaginative resources were critical, but so also necessary were friends. C. J. L., for example, I discovered when he was engaged in a noisy incoherent barrack room argument about Picasso. C. J. L. saw himself as a later day Socrates exposing the ignorance of those around him through his dialectical reasoning, a dangerous practice in the Barrack Room. He was a believer in Nietzsche and fatally, he got me interested in ideas. What was the world about, what was real, how should we live, what was art – suddenly all these questions began to be of vital importance.

Reading became my way of managing the boredom of the work, and the depressing predictability that the institution cultivated. It was not Look and Learn or my Mother's book club, this time I chose very difficult books, and an image of myself as an 'autodidact', or an 'intellectuel manqué', emerged as I embarked on a mission to educate myself. I did not think it was going to be the standard bourgeoise conception of what an education should be, I was afraid that any formal academic task would defeat me and leave me humiliated. I had to find a way of holding on to my phantasy life. This pursuit of enlightenment was not going to be systematic, but, in the spirit of the 1960s, it was going to be a venture that was engaged in doubt, and I had the image of Wilson's (1970) 'Outsider' to inspire me. I tried Sartre's Nausea and Nietszche's Zarathustra and hid Joyce's Ulysses in the drawer of my desk when working in the post office, a place where nothing much seemed to happen, and where it was easy to give the appearance of being busy. You could say that nothing much happens in Ulysses since it focusses on one day in a life, but this imaginative exploration of the mundane inspired me. Limited as my understanding was, difficult texts provided the necessary stimulation for the growth of a precariously independent life, inside, and, through the creation of a fragile imaginary internal world, outside of the institution.

My interest in art was kept alive through drawing and painting but it was difficult to find a space and time for this. I was posted to Germany and there, luckily I found an empty barrack room which the authorities allowed me to use as an 'Art Club', until it was eventually discovered that nobody attended this club, except myself, and a young friend, D., who worked in the NAAFI (shop and café). Mostly the two of us wanted to produce 'modern art' which nobody around us could tolerate. What I produced I later destroyed, but the processes involved seemed to be important to me, and I think to D., although neither of us would have been able to say why.

As a 16-year-old 'boy entrant' I had been obliged to sign on for 9 years plus 3 in the reserves and now, at 20 years, 4 years later, I realised that it was time to get out of the RAF. As a first step, it was necessary to convince the officers that could authorise an application for discharge that I was unhappy and unlikely ever to become the military subject they intended me to be; second, I needed to save money to pay the Royal Air Force some compensation as I was breaking my contract. The first step was not too difficult since a scan of my service record showed that I could be troublesome. I can now proudly report that I had been found guilty of 'conduct prejudicial to good order and Royal Air Force discipline'. The second part took time. However, when the money was accumulated I was told that I would still have to wait until the numbers in my trade group were at a level which would allow for my departure.

There was a long wait, until 1972, which was hard and depressing. In the interim, I studied English and History in the evening Adult Education that the RAF provided. Gaining an A level boosted my confidence and I researched Art Schools and discovered that there was now a possibility of attending an Art School. The Prime Minister Harold Wilson was then enthusiastic for all British Subjects to have access to higher education, if they felt they could benefit from it, and mature student grants were available. Eventually, my depression lifted on one sunny day in May when I was invited to participate in the discharge processes which culminated in handing my uniform into the stores. I think of it now as an exhilarating second birth, and I remember a joyful ride across the flat fens on my motorbike towards Cambridge to begin life as a civilian.

What did I take with me? I had grown submissive and timid in relation to authority and the freedoms of Art School, which although liberating, were often felt as intimidating. There was a call for 'self-expression' and 'spontaneity', in the Art School setting, a demand for a different kind of subject that was difficult for somebody who had become reliant on institutional routine, to meet. The enjoyment of my autodidactic habits did not help. I was required to learn that there were other forms of open enquiry which demanded the use of the hands in interactions with materials. I had some notion of this from my previous efforts at painting and drawing, but now I had to develop a capacity for fresh forms of thinking.

In the RAF I had become aware of social stratification, rank, and the distribution of power. Art schools are also institutions, and I began to think about class, and the relations that contextualised teaching and the production of art and artists – not quite as clearly as this way of remembering suggests. The individual struggling with self-expression and existential 'angst' and 'authenticity' present in Abstract Expressionism was still in the air, and present in the tutor's talk, but I became interested in Marx and student politics, and I began to notice that the Art World itself was producing 'conceptual art'. I wanted to maintain a commitment to modernist painting and wasn't quite ready for discreetly framed typescripts. There were contradictory desires here to manage.

About four years after a postgraduate University course in Fine Art, I joined a project that provided paintings for hospitals in the East End of London. The canvasses, using oil and acrylic, were intended to be traditional perspectival pictures, and we, the artists producing these mural-sized images, were expected to apply the lessons of the 'old masters' to scenes of the East End. On Fridays, we opened our studios to the patients and engaged in conversations and interactions with them. I then began to consider Art Therapy as work. Work, which involves the discipline of repetition and regularity was unwanted, but poverty on a long-term basis was not desirable. Art Therapy was acceptable to the image I then had of myself, and in a cautious and ambivalent manner I approached my training.

Art Therapy training, for me, became a protracted process. There was an initial year, full-time, which lead to a diploma. The experience of working with others in groups, learning to look all over again and to listen, to oneself and others, came as a shock. It was demanding in a way that Art School and University were not. Clinical placements were stressful, but there was some excitement in the air in the institutions in which I worked, which were keen on Art Therapy, and I had a feeling that I was engaged in something of importance. This first year was followed by a part-time course called the Advanced Diploma which I began once I had found work. The course enabled me to digest the experiences had in the initial year. I wanted to challenge myself and I began working with 'Difficult Patients', but the difficulties experienced resulted in self-doubt. In addition to regular support from psychotherapy and clinical supervision, I felt I had to return to the training institution again, to complete an M.A. through part-time study. Slowly I began to recognise that my 'education', or self-awareness, would never be a completed project.

PART 2

N Colony, Becoming Hospital B

From 1913 to 1950

The beginnings of N Colony, later renamed Hospital B, lie in the passing of the Mental Deficiency Act. (1913) (see Wikipedia – Mental Deficiency Act 1913). The bill and the act was passed with only three votes against it. Winston Churchill represented the Eugenicists view which had gained a large following in the House of Commons, he suggested to the Prime Minister in 1910 that the feeble minded should be 'segregated under proper conditions so that the curse died with them and was not transmitted to future generations' (Rutherford 2022 p80). The act was passed in the House of Commons and given Royal Assent in August 1913 'but without enforced sterilisation included' instead 'people deemed undesirable' for instance, 'idiots, feebleminded or moral imbeciles would be separated and isolated from society in institutions'. (Rutherford 2022 p 90).

Drawing on Tredgold's (1908) definitions the act could apply to a range of mental incapacity or deficiency, from 'idiots', 'imbeciles', 'feeble-minded persons' to 'moral imbeciles' (see Chapter 1). The act allowed for parents of 'defective' children who are above the age of 7 years, to petition to have their children admitted to an institution. Such a petition required the support of two qualified medical practitioners and could be originated by other local agents, the courts for instance, other training institutions but also friends or relatives. If the 'defective', once identified, has been abandoned and neglected and has no visible means of support; if about to be sent to an industrial school; if in imprisonment; if habitually drunk; if found in a criminal lunatic asylum; or if in receipt of poor relief at the time of giving birth to an illegitimate child, then a petition might be made and approved. Being 'defective' indicated an inability to fulfil a function, a function determined by social stratification. The act identifies a large heterogeneous portion of the population who were not considered capable of fulfilling their 'duties' as Tredgold put it. Instead, this group was often destitute and dependent on others.

World War I delayed the implementation of this act and it was not until 1928 that County Councils began to invest in, and build the 'rural colonies', as the required total institutions were first called. All colonies were intended to provide a sheltered and segregated environment at a distance from any town, in a rural location, where fresh air and wholesome food and exercise were available. Isolation was intended to prevent any 'moral contagion', but the result in relation to family relations was not good; visits were especially difficult for poorer families, in effect 'defectives' were incarcerated and abandoned to live in the colony – thus achieving the segregation that the Eugenicists desired.

Labour, work and/or training, was central to the colony idea. The colony, which later became hospital B, I shall call 'N' Colony. It was first inhabited by 'higher grade mental defectives' and their 'attendants' – the staff who lived in the colony. The attendant's role was custodial as well as disciplinary in relation to work tasks.

Residents, were to be escorted at all times by attendants who operated a locked environment and carried keys. Attendants were gradually replaced by nurses as the diversity of the population increased.

A central administration building was built, and on one side of the central road villas for male residents, and on the opposite side villas for female residents. The separation between men and women was 'strictly enforced' and a boundary line was used to mark out the two territories. As well as the villas there were pavilions that housed the physically disabled, those regarded as 'low grade', and those needing some nursing care. Accommodation for nursing staff was built and the Medical Superintendent was housed in a farmhouse. Places and spaces indicated clearly the gender and class relations that structured this community.

Two farms were established on the site, and the patients or residents were involved in farming activities, rearing cattle, pigs and chickens, growing fruit and vegetables and producing milk. Workshops included tailoring, shoe-making, brush-making, carpentry and upholstery. Women were mostly employed in the laundry, in the kitchens that supplied the villas, and in scrubbing floors. Employed is the word used in the Hospital History, but this is not the right word here, because residents did not receive any wages, instead they were gifted with pocket money or cigarettes for 'good work' and 'good behaviour', and as a resident recalls, in the Hospital History, 'the nurses were very strict then'.

The idea of leisure was not neglected both in relation to the staff and the residents themselves. A hall, named after the County Alderman was erected and this was equipped with a stage for amateur dramatics, and much later, in the 1960s provided with cinema equipment. Dancing was allowed in the hall but not between *residents* of the opposite sex. N colony also had its own mortuary and sick ward.

The colony did become self-sufficient and surpluses, from the farms and the workshops, were sold to nearby markets, until, in the late 1930s local traders opposed this. In time some residents were 'licensed' to work outside. Whether they were properly paid or not we do not know.

In the 1930s, the Eugenics Society became concerned that ineffective environmental, or social measures aimed at 'defectives' would end in the 'proliferation' of 'the unfit' (Bland and Hall 2010). There were fresh calls for voluntary and/or compulsory sterilisation and the Minister of Health created a departmental committee to examine the issue and report to Parliament. This resulted in the Brock report of 1934 which provides a clear picture of contemporary thinking in relation to 'mental deficiency'.

The report opens by indicating that it was important to examine sterilisation as a preventative measure in relation to mental defectiveness, as there were, 'serious social results' and the likelihood of 'moral corruption' should there be a failure 'to control the mental defective' (p5).

The report begins by considering the evidence for heredity transmission and other environmental causes of defectiveness. Dr Penrose and Dr Turner who examined 513 patients in institutional settings and studied family histories, supplied the committee with medical evidence that showed hereditary causation to be present amongst 29% of their sample, and that there was evidence for environmental causation in relation to the 'lower grades' of defective. However, the committee took the view that intelligence was largely inherited and that 'feeblemindedness was definitely inherited'.

There was considerable anxiety, expressed in the report, concerning a further group present in the 'lower social stratum'. The report argued that there was no clear 'line of cleavage' between 'dullness' and the 'higher grade mental defective' and that mental defect was able to perpetuate itself 'by creating an environment inimical to the development of normal mentality' (p54).

> We [the committee] were impressed by the dead weight of social inefficiency and individual misery which is entailed by the existence within our midst of over a quarter of a million mental defectives and of a larger number of persons who without being certifiably defective are mentally subnormal.
>
> (p55)

Presumably this other 'mentally subnormal' group, who have not been certified, are the 'dull' group who are close to the feeble minded from the 'lower social stratum', and who are held responsible, along with the 'feeble minded', for a degraded environment, and 'the dead weight of social inefficiency'.

The committee did not think that there was any 'wholesale racial deterioration' but they did think that the number of 'defectives and subnormals' was 'probably growing'. Segregation was the solution to the problems identified, voluntary sterilisation, with safeguards in relation to consent, could be practiced, but compulsory sterilisation was not recommended. There was no evidence provided for holding that 'defectives and subnormals' were responsible for the production of the toxic environmental conditions from which they suffered, and neither was the committee particularly clear in respect of the threat of a 'moral corruption' that this group seemed to personify, especially as they found that the 'supposed abnormal fertility' of defectives was 'mythical' (Brock 1934, p38).

The anxieties evident in the report should be understood in the context of the social and political instabilities present in the 1930s, where unemployment and poverty were widespread. The departmental committee's report was indicating that the social ills that they have identified could only be generated by those sections of the working classes, the 'dull' and 'subnormal' that were in the 1930s facing widespread destitution, because of situations in which they had little in the way of power to affect.

A Scout Troop and a band of bugles and drums were formed in N colony in the 1930s. In 1939 the nation faced other, external, threats. Once the war had begun there were staff shortages. However, residents continued to demonstrate their productivity, in the farm and in the workshops, and in addition, helping other local farms with harvests, and this was now appreciated as a contribution to the war effort.

Hospital B from 1950 to 1989

In 1950 the N Colony was renamed Hospital B as it passed from the control of the county council to the newly formed National Health Service. Nursing training was now emphasised and a move 'from the status of warder-like attendants to professional registered nurses was required. Unfortunately recruitment difficulties arose because of the isolation of the hospital. The problem was addressed through the building of more nursing accommodation and recruitment from overseas, and nurses came from Ireland, Italy, Spain, Mauritius, the West Indies, the Indian sub-continent, West Africa and the Far East (Hospital History).

The 1950s saw a change in the discursive environment. Medical practices, in relation to the 'defective', became more sharply focussed on genetics; but there were also attempts to treat mental abnormality through surgery – often with very unhappy results. More significantly the 1950s saw the rise of behavioural psychology, and cognitive psychology, and psychologists working with institutional populations began researching mental deficiency. O'Connor and Tizard (1956), for example, wanted to demonstrate that as a result of behavioural forms of instruction and education, 'detained defectives' were able to work in open employment and/or in sheltered facilities and that behavioural methodologies were capable of 'turning out socially competent citizens' (p7).

Cognitive psychologists were interested in assessing intelligence and in identifying developmental levels. They introduced fresh categorisations of 'defectiveness' and directed their activities towards remedial interventions which would be individually tailored. 'Ineducable' became a term in use alongside the use of subnormal and severely subnormal. However in the report of the Royal Commission on the Law related to Mental Illness and Mental Deficiency which reported to Parliament in 1957 'defective' was still the preferred term. The report recognised that an individual could be both 'defective and disordered' and it argues that a 'Lack of intelligence' does not by itself indicate mental defection: 'it is only when arrested or incomplete mental development (which may include lack of intelligence) makes a person incapable of managing without special care that he is regarded as mentally defective' (HMSO 1957, p27).

The report with its emphasis on development, and the individual's capacity, or incapacity, for 'managing' his or herself, without care in the community, represents an endorsement of the approach favoured by cognitive and behavioural psychologists.

The report resulted in the 1959 Mental Health Act, a replacement for the act of 1913. The act required Local Authorities to provide training and social care in the community and to provide 'occupational centres' for adult defectives. Parents could seek an admission to hospitals through an application to specially appointed Justices of the Peace, and under the act admissions for defectives, defined as a 'subject to be dealt with', could take place. Admissions were not intended to be long term and were expected to be reviewed regularly (HMSO 1960). In 1961, Enoch

Powell, then Minister of Health called for all Mental Health Hospitals, whether for defective or disordered patients to close within 15 years (Open University 2022).

It is odd that behavioural psychologists felt the need to research the question of employment to *demonstrate* that 'defectives' were capable, with instruction and support, of being productive. The history of the hospital, or N Colony as it was once called, clearly shows that in terms of farming, tailoring, shoe making and repair, brush making, carpentry and laundry their achievements were impressive. However, during the 1960s and 1970s, it was 'Occupational and Industrial Therapy' which dominated practices. This resulted in patients losing work opportunities that were of benefit to the hospital community. These were now being taken on by 'domestic staff'. Not surprisingly there was some 'resentment amongst the residents'; 'Where else would I get a job like this?' said S. a resident working as supervisor in the wine-making section (Hospital History). Of course had S. a job in Wine Making outside of the hospital setting, he would have been paid properly, as well.

During the 1950s and 1960s Hospital B made contracts with local commercial firms for assembly and packing of toys and games and the manufacture of chain link fencing. 'Younger male residents with behavioural disorders' experienced 'work discipline' in 'the manufacture of concrete slabs and posts', we are told, but 'there were no strict production targets' (Hospital History). If others were making gains from the unpaid labour of the residents, the hospital saw this different form of work as therapeutic, and the previous active self-sufficiency as regressive.

The 1960s and the 1970s saw the expansion of services; a Cerebral Palsy Unit, new physiotherapy services, and the development of new treatments for deaf-blind children. Resident children were taught at a school attached to the Hospital, administered by the Local Authority. The Occupational Therapy Unit introduced crafts, rug-making, knitting, embroidery and pottery to residents as a 'multi-disciplinary approach to patient care' was encouraged. The new psychology department focussed on 'behaviour modification' and the hospital offered this service to local adult training centres.

The 'L M' Centre was opened in 1965 and remained attached to the Hospital until 1987. A major focus of research in this centre was on the prenatal diagnosis of chromosomal abnormalities in the foetus. Positively the Professor Director of this centre insisted that 'research and treatment should be complementary' and the Psychology Department did, in response, create an 'experimental' playgroup (Hospital History).

Overcrowding at Hospital B became a problem in the 1960s as admissions increased. Despite the call for community care present in the 1959 act and the following call from the Minister for Health, for the closure of large long-stay hospitals, many large hospitals grew in size. In the 1970s there were many hospital scandals. In Somerset, Lancashire, Hertfordshire and Essex there were reports of corruption, poor quality of care, violence and mistreatment. In the south of the country, in

1976, the Confederation of Health Service Employees (COHSE) took strike action because they argued that the management was attempting to block justified complaints in relation to poor care – this resulted in a public inquiry which concluded that Senior Medical, nursing and admin staff were failing to co-operate with each other (Rivett 1998).

In the late 1970s, after the scandals, there was a move to return, where possible, residents to the community from which they originated, and the hospital population did then begin to decrease, but progress in this direction was slow. The Hospital History reported that some older patients died, but those remaining 'tended to be more difficult to place'.

In 1980 the preferred term for the hospital population became People with Mental Handicap, replacing the deficiency labels that had been in use previously. People with Learning Difficulties was the term adopted by self-advocacy groups in 1985 and, in 1990, by the Department of Health (Open University 2022). A white paper, Caring for People: Community Care in the next Decade and Beyond was produced in 1989 calling for the procurement of care services, including residential care, by the local government. It called for People with Learning Difficulties to be living at home, where possible. There was a call for the reduction of costs to the Department of Social Security and it was suggested that funds, which were now expected to be provided by Local Government, should be directed towards those with the greatest need. The white paper also sought to promote the growth of the independent sector in providing care, which brings in the profit motive (Department of Health & Department of Social Security 1989).

I Arrive at Hospital B

I arrived at hospital B in 1989, and at that time, there were 750 residents living in the hospital. As the hospital was focussed on closing and finding community placements for all residents, there were to be no more admissions, except for small numbers of short-term patients/residents to the admissions and treatment service. As community placement involved the identification of funding from local authorities progress remained slow. Psychiatrists and psychologists who worked in the hospital were now closely linked to the communities that the hospital served. Everything was orientated towards outside and workshops were gradually closing.

Art Therapy was introduced to the hospital in 1977. My predecessor worked in a room next door to the physiotherapists. Some money had been provided by a voluntary group linked to the hospital for the provision of facilities, and it was decided that the old mortuary could be converted into an Art Therapy Department and a Speech and Language Department. The hospital had maintained a sick ward, but the mortuary was closed in the 1960s.

In the mortuary, autopsies were undertaken and specimens collected; there was also storage facility and a Chapple of Rest. Pathological anatomy was regarded as important to the research which was focussed on the 'defective'. It was capable of

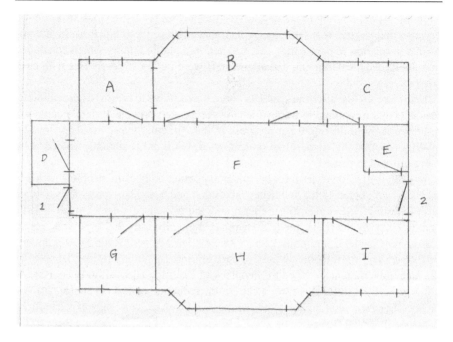

Figure 2 A sketch of the Art Therapy Department as I remember it.

disclosing disease and impairment and autopsies could provide specimens and add to the number of known cases.

In Figure 2 you can see the layout of the mortuary after conversion into the two departments, Art Therapy, and Speech and Language Therapy.

A = Art Therapy Office, formally the specimens room.
B = Art Therapy Room for Group and Individual Work, formally the room where autopsies were undertaken.
C = Smaller Art Therapy Space for Individual Work, formally storage facility.
D = Toilet.
E = Toilet for Wheel-Chair users.
F = Corridor.
G = Speech and Language Therapy Office.
H = Speech and Language Therapy Large Room, mostly used as a waiting area, formally Chapple of Rest.
I = Small Speech and Language Room for Individual Work.
1 – Main Entrance, and 2 – Fire door and exit.

In the original design for the Art Therapy Department, a small observation window with mirror glass on one side was to be inserted in the wall between the Art

Therapy Office and the Large Therapy Room (A and B in the sketch), and microphones attached to the centre of the ceiling in B, were linked to recording equipment in the office A.

The idea that individuals could be assessed through the examination of behaviour had been around since the 1950s, and this emphasis on surveillance and recording, in the design, could be understood as a continuation of the research practices of the experimental playgroups of the 1960s. Via the conversion, the previous anatomy of corpses had been translated into an anatomy of behaviour.

Ironically some strange coincidental mis-communication was at work during the building of the Speech and Language and Art Therapy Departments, and the dimensions for the 'small' observation window with mirror glass was enlarged by the builders so that the window almost covered the whole of the wall from floor to ceiling and side to side. The microphones never functioned properly, and no attempt was made to correct this. I covered the large window/mirror with a curtain and did not use the microphones. However, observation and assessment became a task that was attached to my role. As well as working on the hospital site, my predecessor worked at 'Chestnut House' an Edwardian Building close to the hospital that provided a multi-disciplinary assessment service for Children and Young People who were thought to have Neuro-developmental Disorders. Here the use of video cameras was in regular use, and I too was obliged to navigate this practice (see Chapter 2). This use of video did play into my practice, in the sense that I optimistically believed that I could know a subject through careful observation.

The early 1980s saw the beginnings of the development of a social model of disability (Oliver 1986, 1990) which gave emphasis to the difference between an impairment and a disability which was understood as socially produced. Psychoanalytical psychotherapy for children and adults with Learning Disabilities was provided by the Tavistock Clinic during the 1980s and, as this work was now being researched and publicised (see Sinason 1992), a small number of staff in Hospital B developed a desire to shift practices towards a more psychoanalytical understanding of subjectivity and identity. In thinking about my own practices I wanted to provide a therapeutic intervention, using art-making, that offered a different kind of experience. Would it be possible to create a setting that benefits both, the resident, and the therapist, where both learn from the other?

Before we look at what was possible in the following chapters I want to provide something that communicates the emotional atmosphere of the context that I have been trying to describe.

During my first two weeks at work in Hospital B, I visited the wards, not only to introduce myself to the nursing staff but also to gain some sense of the life of the 'residents' (the preferred term within the hospital). I entered ward number 13 'Green Pastures' and I was greeted by the ward manager. He was happy to introduce himself and show me around the ward. We entered the dining area. The dining area was prepared for tea and the return of the residents from workshops and day centres. Small Formica topped tables were arranged uniformly in rows spreading across the floor of the square room, which had dull yellow ochre walls. As the late afternoon light streamed in from the windows I could see dust slowly falling onto the individual place settings, the knives and forks, the table surface, and, more poignant, falling gently onto the soft white bread slices that had been carefully placed on small plates next to the cutlery. This scene immediately prompted sad recollections of other experiences, of life in another 'total institution'. Here was an unwelcome return to my institutional home.

References

Bland, L. & Hall, L. A. 2010. Eugenics in Britain: The View from the Metropolis. In: Bashford, A. & Levine, P. (Eds.) *The Oxford Handbook of the History of Eugenics.* Oxford University Press, Oxford, pp. 213–227.

Brock, L. G. 1934. *Brock Report of the Departmental Committee on Sterilization.* HM Stationery Office, London.

Butler, J. 1997. *The Psychic Life of Power – Theories in Subjection.* Stanford University Press, Stanford.

Department of Health & Department of Social Security. 1989. *Caring for People, Community Care in the Next Decade and Beyond.* Her Majesties Stationery Office, London.

Foucault, M. 1991. *Discipline and Punish – The Birth of the Prison.* Sheridan, A. (Trans.). Penguin Books. London, New York, Victoria Australia, Ontario Canada, New Delhi, Auckland New Zealand, & Rosebank South Africa.

Foucault, M. 2002. The Subject and Power. In: Faubion, J. D. (Ed.) and Hurley, R. et al. (Trans.) *Michel Foucault – Power – Essential Works of Foucault 1954–1984*, Volume 3. Penguin Books. London, New York, Victoria Australia, Ontario Canada, New Delhi, Auckland New Zealand, & Rosebank South Africa, pp. 326–348.

Goffman, E. 1987. *Asylums – Essays on the Social Situation of Mental Patients and Other Inmates.* Peregrine Books – Penguin Books, London.

HMSO. 1957. *Royal Commission on the Law Related to Mental Illness and Mental Deficiency.* Her Majesties Stationery Office, London, available at: http://wellcomecollection.org.

HMSO. 1960. *Mental Health Act 1959.* Her Majesties Stationery Office, London, available at: http://wellcomecollection.org.

Mental Deficiency Act. 1913. Education in England – 2 Nov 2019, available at: http://www.educationengland.org.uk. See also Wikipedia on the Parliamentary Debate.

O'Connor, N. & Tizard, J. 1956. *The Social Problem of Mental Deficiency.* Pergamon Press, Oxford.

Oliver, M. 1986. Social Policy and Disability: Some Theoretical Issues, *Disability, Handicap & Society* 1(1): 5–18.

Oliver, M. 1990. *The Politics of Disablement.* Macmillan, London.

Open University. 2022. *Timeline of Learning Disability History/Social History of Learning Disability.* Accessed via the Open University Website: open.ac.uk

Rivett, G. 1998. *From the Cradle to the Grave: The History of the NHS 1948–1987.* The King's Fund, London.

Rutherford, A. 2022. *Control – The Dark History and Troubling Present of Eugenics.* Weidenfeld & Nicolson, London.

Sinason, V. 1992. *Mental Handicap and the Human Condition – New Approaches from the Tavistock.* Free Association Books, London.

Tredgold, A. F. 1908. *Mental Deficiency (Amentia).* Bailliere, Tindall and Cox, London. Covent Garden – Digitized by the Internet Archive in 2016. https://archive.org/details/b28047667 – accessed 08.08.22.

Mental Deficiency Act 1913. Wikipedia – accessed Sep 2023.

Wilson, C. 1970. *The Outsider.* Pan Books Ltd., London.

Chapter 4

Amy

Introduction

This case study, I would like to think of as a case his/herstory, since it is *my* story, made according to my reading of the hospital documents, the notes that I made at the time, my view of Amy's art work, and my subsequent interpretation and reflections; and *Amy's* story insofar as I have remembered her speech and her activity in Art Therapy, and in so far as I have been able to present Amy's art production as self-expression and communication. I wanted it to be a his/herstory because I wanted to remember Amy, who I was and where I was, and I wanted others to picture a therapeutic couple, and imagine the life Amy lead in hospital B.

Amy was 62 years old when she began her Art Therapy. She had lived for 45 years in hospital B. Hospital documents indicated that she was born with Spina Bifida. They record that Amy spoke at 2 years of age. She did not walk until 3 years of age and the right side of her body, in particular her right arm, were attenuated and lacked the strength of her left side and arm. These physical differences were not obvious from her appearance. Amy attended school until the age of 13 years and then, presumably because of her poor performance at school, and difficulties at home, she was regarded as having a learning disability, and was referred by the National Provisional Council for Mental Welfare, in May 1944, to Estuary Valley Institution. She was resident in this institution for four years and then transferred to Hospital B.

Amy is described in the documents as an individual who found it difficult to complete simple tasks; for example when washing her face she stops and starts washing the wall. She locked herself into the toilet on occasions, was also incontinent at times (incontinence is often present with spina bifida), and could be aggressive to others, it is reported. At 54 years of age, Amy was scored on the Wechsler Adult Intelligence Scales as follows: Verbal 63, Performance 58 and Full Score 58. The psychologist commented that she 'appears to understand and retain verbal instructions but fails to behave according to them'. This is similar to a comment made in the nursing notes where it is written, 'has continually to be told what, and when to do things'.

Amy referred herself to Art Therapy. She saw me one day when I visited the ward to talk to another resident and, since I was new to her, she decided to follow

DOI: 10.4324/9781003360056-5

me to see where I came from. Amy then came into the department and asked if she could come to Art Therapy. I tried to explain to Amy what she might expect if she attended for Art Therapy, for example, that I saw art making as a way of exploring problems, and I asked again if she still wished to come. 'Yes', she said, and asked if she would get a cup a tea in the department. I did say that she could have tea at the end of the session, and I agreed to check with the ward staff and others who cared for her and, providing they thought it was OK, she could come to Art Therapy. I felt at the end of this exchange that Amy had charmed me, with her smile, smart appearance, and her direct questions, into offering her my services. The ward staff told me that it was planned for Amy to be moved on to live in the community. A placement had not been identified and it was thought that it could take some time. Amy, they felt, could make good use of Art Therapy as a support during the resettlement process.

Amy clearly enjoyed the conversation. She was popular and well-known amongst the staff and residents of the hospital. What I quickly learned was that, although Amy appeared to chatter away in a trivial fashion, jumping from subject to subject, she was in fact very adept at asking questions and ferreting out information, and, during our first encounter, I felt sure that Amy was making a careful assessment of me.

Narrative and Reflection

First Session

Amy wanted to know all about me. She also wanted to know what had happened to my predecessor whom she had seen for three sessions. I told Amy that she had moved to another hospital to work. I then suggested to Amy that we should meet for a trial period of ten weeks to see if she could make use of Art Therapy. I pointed towards the art materials, explaining what was available for use and I indicated that when she had produced some work we could look at it and think about it together, and that this process could be a way of thinking about problems. Amy remained standing near to the table, while I was seated nearer to the door.

Amy wanted to paint, and painted while standing. She said that she liked 'mauve' but that this was a colour that her mother did not like. With the 'mauve' paint she produced a house, and below a figure which, Amy proposed, 'could be me' (Figure 3).

I pointed to the absence of a door, not immediately thinking that this might be received critically, but rather thinking that this absence might, in itself, be an important communication. Amy said that she had forgot, but then added there was not enough room between the windows. She then added a door. Amy then talked about theft by other residents and murderers outside the hospital. She said that there was a story in the newspaper about a baby being badly treated. I commented that she thought that people did some bad things 'stealing, murder, and badly treating babies' and that made her feel anxious in here – in the department.

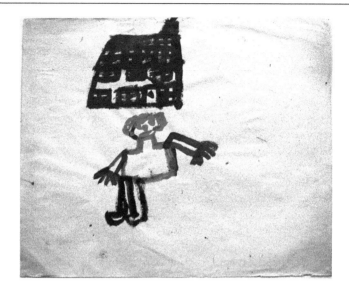

Figure 3 House and Figure. Tempera paint on A2.

The 'mauve' house refers to home and to her mother. Amy wants the therapist to know that her tastes are her own, independent of her mother's preferences. The house appears just above the head of the figure which, judging by size, stands at some distance from the house. The figure is painted in a range of colours, a bright orange-red for the head, neck, shoulders and right side of torso, whilst two blues are used for the arms and torso, and a dark red to outline legs and feet. All this gives an emphasis to its composition from parts. The left arm of the figure is larger than the right, which could reflect Amy's body dysmorphia, and this would then be a reference to spina-bifida.

My comment about the absent door does now appear to me to be clumsy. Amy stresses that there was, with this house, insufficient space for the door and squeezes one in, to satisfy the therapist. Amy is thereby stressing the painting process, and excusing a perceived failure, but I am thinking in a Freudian frame, that 'mistakes', and forgetting have a significance. If this really is a message about the difficulty of gaining entrance to this house, or home, then it is the possibility of a home, that might be denied her. It is, for sure, her mother and herself that Amy presents in her painting as her preoccupation, her 'problem'.

Second Session

Amy arrived late for the second session. She told me that she had spent 'a long time over breakfast'. She again asked lots of questions. She asked about my father, was he still alive? I told her that he was dead and then she told me about the death of her parents. She was sorry when her father died but not when her mother died. Her mother, Amy said, neglected her brother who died of T. B. She then told me that she had spina bifida and was worried about Oedema. Amy referred to her mental state and described herself as 'not backward, but not forward, but not a wide-head, but not bright'.

While standing and talking Amy took up the clay and began modelling it. She talked of making a dog and a cat, but she instead made 'balls' and an 'animal or bird' of some kind to which she added eyes. Finally, the whole was turned into 'sausages'.

Her late arrival, and a 'long time over breakfast', suggest that she is unsure about her day and needs some time to make a decision in relation to Art Therapy. There were lots of questions and my brief personal disclosure did appear to help her give an insightful account of herself. She is worried about her health (oedema) and she has lost her parents and a younger brother. Her mother is blamed for this loss. Not being 'backward' or 'forward', nor having a 'wide-head', 'but not being bright' Amy differentiates herself from other residents in the hospital, grading her mental state using the language that she has absorbed from her interactions with others in the institution. The modelling with the clay, in its continuous transformations, suggested to me that I could anticipate further indecision and uncertainty. I am now thinking that in standing, which became a regular feature in her sessions, Amy placed her eye level on the same level as mine. There was something assertive about her gaze and this stance. I also became aware of how disjointed and rapid her speech could be, speech which was accompanied by gesture and movement as she contemplated the clay on the table before her. I felt that I was going to fail to note all that was said, that it was going to require attentiveness and patience to capture the important communications.

Third Session

On arrival Amy asked 'Why didn't I give her tea?' I responded with 'I'm not giving you what you need'. Amy said 'That's right not giving me what I need'. In a more interpretative mode, I suggested, 'Maybe you feel empty inside and you want me to take away the empty feeling'. Amy said, 'Yes I'm empty inside'. This was said without any sign of affect; perhaps she understood my comment literally. Amy then talked of 'rows' with her boyfriend, and with the nurse 'nagging'. As she spoke, she was drawing circles, apples and a box. The nurse, she, said 'Kept asking if I was going or not' (to the Art Therapy department).

*I had agreed with Amy that she could have tea at the end of the session when she referred herself to Art Therapy and Amy probably felt, rightly, that I had not kept my word. I had not yet organised a kettle etc. and I should have said 'I am not giving you what was agreed'. The tea was part of the exchange, she used the materials, and provided me with an object of visual interest, in return I would provide tea. Why would any resident in the hospital visit any department if they did not provide tea? The not giving tea was an expression of **my** ambivalence. The nurse was clearly aware of Amy's ambivalence but Amy needs time to decide if Art Therapy is* *worthwhile, or indeed if a relationship with this therapist will be worthwhile, will there simply be 'rows' or 'nagging' and no tea.*

Fourth Session

I told Amy that I would be away the following week as it was Whitsun, and this was a staff holiday. She spoke again about tea, 'You don't make tea, A used to' She was referring to my predecessor who she had seen for three sessions. 'Is that a kettle up there?' she asked. She then talked about the cruelty of staff which then lead her on to suggest that dogs and cats were dangerous, 'a cat suffocated somebody' she concluded. I said that she could draw a dog and/or a cat. She decided instead to draw 'boxes' and a 'bird'. This was followed by a chair and a table with five legs. Looking up towards where the kettle was, she commented that 'other patients would smash that cup, I wouldn't'. I suggested that she could be angry about the holiday I was taking. She agreed that she was and then she remembered her Dad dying and said that her brother would not have her at home.

Still no tea and now a holiday! I have the kettle and cups – what's missing now, tea, milk? The battle is between staff and residents, perhaps dogs and cats. She restrains herself and does not smash the cup, and is able to recognise her feelings, feelings principally about the staff who do not deliver their part of the agreement, and who take holidays. This brings her father and her brother to mind. I was left wondering about the boxes and the bird, and why a table might require five legs.

Fifth Session

Amy came late and said, 'didn't want to come really'. She had also bought her friend Barry along with her, and he waited in the corridor. Amy referred to the bank holiday, saying that bank holiday Monday means missing a session. I pointed out that I did offer her an extra session on the Wednesday, but she did not take up that offer. She said, 'I did want to come and I didn't, it sounds silly really doesn't it'. I suggested that she found it difficult here. 'I do but I want to come' she responded.

Amy acknowledges her ambivalence, but she reassures me that she does want to come. She introduces me to Barry, letting me know that she has a male friend, and that there are other relationships in her life. I needed to make up my mind.

Sixth Session

Amy began by telling me that she wet the bed, really because she was too lazy to get out. She then talked about a 'resident' whose brother did not visit although this resident believed that her brother was going to take her out. She then suggested that her brother was like me. I then asked if she thought that I had let her down. 'Yes when you went on holiday', she said. I then suggested that she was both angry and sad. But Amy responded with, 'You say I am but how do you know how I feel?'. And with some passion, she then talked of wanting to get out of here. She didn't like the staff and the food was 'shit'. She then apologised for the swearing, 'I shouldn't have said that should I?'.

She wanted to use the clay, but her hand was hovering, for a long time, over a lump, that I had placed on the table. Maybe, I was thinking to myself, she felt it was 'shit', like my interpretative comment about her feelings. Eventually she sliced the lump into two halves. I said 'maybe that is how you feel today, one half wanting to use the materials, one half not'. Amy responded to this comment, 'It is true isn't it – yes I suppose I am like that'.

*Incontinence often goes with spina – bifida but she confesses to being lazy. Was I going to let her down, like her brother, are my materials 'shit'? Of course, she is right, I do not know how she feels, in the sense that I cannot fully experience her feelings, after all **she** is the one that has to live her life in the hospital, when she is desperate to leave. I do experience Amy's feelings when they are expressed by expletives and her actions with the clay, and some agreement about feeling at the end of the session was reached.*

Seventh Session

Amy spent ten minutes in the toilet before coming into the therapy room. She talked about Church ornaments and death, the death of a patient, this was followed by an account of a mother who threw her baby over the cliff (this was on TV) and then she told me that her mother and father neglected her brother. She then said how she was missing tea in the canteen. I then agreed that she could have tea here at the end of the session, I would make some. She then produced a drawing of a 'square box' which had a cross on it.

The time in the toilet seemed to be a way of approaching the session slowly, by degrees, maintaining autonomy whilst making a decision. Her brother who died, was, Amy suggests, neglected by a murderous mother, as well as her father. This brother, and the neglect, was first mentioned in the second session. I was wondering about the baby being 'thrown over the cliff'. 'Thrown over' suggests an abandonment, a murderous abandonment. We now have tea. Maybe this is my way of saying that I will not be a murderous or neglectful parent, and that I am committed to the relationship. The box, like the earlier boxes and apples left me puzzled. The cross on the box seems to seal it in some way. Perhaps our deal has been sealed as I am now delivering tea.

Eighth Session

In the Eighth session Amy asked, 'When will I meet your wife?' She drew boxes which she said had something inside, but that she didn't know what. She also drew apples but was uncertain of where to place the stalks. Then we were disturbed by Barry who was in the corridor and he wanted to say goodbye to Amy. He kissed her goodbye and left. I said, 'you wanted me to see that somebody cares for you'. She said 'Yes'.

Amy wants to know who cares for me. Or now it's time to meet the family. Since I have met Barry she should meet my wife. Apples and boxes appeared in the third session. The boxes are mysterious in relation to their insides. I am now inclined to associate the boxes and the apples with knowledge of some kind, a sexual awareness, and she is thinking about relations between men and women in this session. Maybe they are ballot boxes, since they can be sealed, and Amy wants to know if she gets my vote.

Ninth Session

Amy told me that her head was spinning round. During the session she was dropping off to sleep and waking up, and dropping off again. She asked if I had any tea things and I made her tea. I asked at the end of the session if the things that I say make her head spin round. 'Yes' was the answer.

The spinning head and fatigue may be related to her oedema, a sign of some heart or circulatory problem. I didn't think this at the time. But I was surprised by her sleepiness, and I was concerned that perhaps Amy was not as robust as I imagined her to be. Her sleeping and my making tea feel like a regression of some sort. Amy needs looking after.

Tenth Session

Amy said that she wasn't well 'last week'. Amy used oil pastels and she drew a house beginning with the roof (Figure 4). She asked 'did you see Sons and Lovers? – the father gave the mother a heart attack and the son left his girlfriend in the end'. Amy added a white door to her house drawing. It was difficult to see it on the white paper. She then drew a bird saying; 'is it a swallow, or is it a yellow hammer? – it's a yellow hammer' (Figure 4).

I reminded Amy that this was the tenth session and the end of the trial period that we had agreed on, and I asked her, 'do you get anything from coming?' A rather strange question in a way, but I suppose I wanted it to be open ended. Amy replied 'a cup of tea'. I then asked, 'does it help you to come?' She replied, 'Yes, I think it helps me do you?' When I asked if she wanted to continue she said, 'I do and I don't'. We then agreed to continue to meet regularly, but that she would have the option of ending at any point if she chose to.

This drawing when related to the first picture of the house in the first session illustrates a development. The figure outside the house has changed into a bird. This large bird has a rectangular crest on the top of its head and an almost human face, the bill or beak has the appearance of an open and empty mouth – not unlike a nestling awaiting feeding. In relation to the house my attention has been drawn to the door again, this time the door is drawn with a white pastel on white paper making it difficult to find or to see clearly.

'Sons and Lovers' is presented as a family drama and Amy has begun to seek an understanding of her own family experiences, but could she have some other

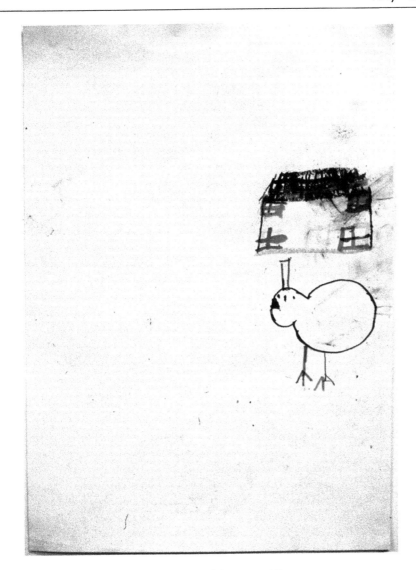

Figure 4 House and bird. Oil pastel and felt tip on A3.

Father in mind? This father gives the mother a heart attack, and what about the son who leaves his girlfriend in the end? The conversation about the value of Art Therapy was a difficult one to have and my initial question did not help. The words 'anything from coming' imply that I had some ambivalent feelings about the value of the therapy. Despite this, her answer was positive in relation to 'help' but she remains in an 'I do and I don't' place which is maybe where the 'yellow hammer' bird is. I think I could have been affirmative in relation to her question, did I think that Art Therapy helped her. Amy's 'do you?' I did not respond to.

Eleventh Session

Amy came late and asked me about the forthcoming bank holiday and wanted to know if she should come on Wednesday. I said Yes, but I would need to confirm by checking my diary at the end of the session. Amy then proceeded to explore her relationship to her two brothers. One brother visits over the holiday and one doesn't. The one who stays away sends a card. Amy complained about him several times, 'he puts love on the card'. She was, she told me, angry with both brothers. The one who visits tells her to 'stop messing around' as, she explained, she goes to the toilet when he arrives on the ward and stays there. She then asked if I am ever angry. I reminded her of being late today and I related this to her feelings and her behaviour towards her brother. After some difficulty in choosing materials Amy composed from paint and charcoal, and said, 'a box with stripes on – shall I put a lid on?' At the end of the session I confirmed that she could come on Wednesday.

The hospital file did not tell me anything about Amy's family, for example the dates of her parent's deaths etc. Maybe I was not looking in the right file but Amy had three brothers, one of whom died. As she tells me in this session of the two remaining brothers only one visits, the other sends a card. Amy is very clear in relation to her anger and the steps she takes to express her feelings. The 'messing around', her behaviour, might also relate to her feelings about bank holidays. Bank holidays are an example of the staff messing around. The 'box' could be regarded as a place where feelings can be contained, where she can, if she wishes, keep 'a lid on' it.

Twelfth Session

Amy told me immediately that her brother visited and she 'told him off'. 'He ought to live here – it's alright for him – what's good for the goose is good for the gander' she continued. She appeared to be happy that she had been able to be angry with him in a direct way and began drawing shapes. She drew circles, squares, diamonds, triangles and stars. She said that there was a patient angry with her at breakfast, and this patient said that she (Amy) should be given 'beetles' for breakfast. Amy thought that this was horrible and went on to tell me that the French eat frogs and snails. She then related how a patient 'fed up with life' ate frogs, and when she died her stomach was found to be 'full of frogs'. Next she told me a story about a man who was hunted because he was a 'poisoner'. He was hung eventually and Amy laughed at this idea. She then, more seriously, asked about 'purgatory – after death', what was 'purgatory' she asked. I did my best to explain what I thought purgatory was and she told me that she was confident of going to heaven. Her shapes were then completed with a star (Figure 5).

Amy's geometry shows Amy to be uncertain. She is maybe struggling to place her lines confidently, some lines and half-formed shapes seem to be beginnings. But I would argue that she wants to be decisive, to see things clearly, to demonstrate that she can remember and reproduce the lessons she has learned, both in terms

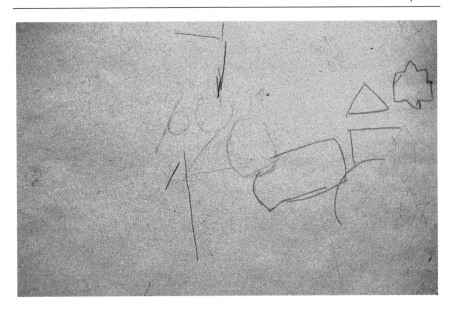

Figure 5 Geometric shapes. Crayon and felt tip on A3.

of geometry and her feelings and experiences – with her brother for instance. The star, bottom right is related to her certainty of going to heaven.

Amy was triumphant at the beginning of the session. 'What's good for the goose is good for the gander' indicates that as she is the recipient of her brother's feeling he can be a recipient of her feeling – it's an equality between the sexes. We know who the patient that is 'fed up with life' is, and this story suggests that she may, in self-hatred, be filling her stomach with suspect foreign food. The French man or other, if I were to interpret with the transference in mind, is a possible threat, and Amy should, therefore, take care of what she swallows, what she takes inside, since there are poisoners around. The stomach full of frogs at the moment of death is indicative of the indigestible nature of some food.

I missed an opportunity to explore Amy's thinking about 'purgatory' by treating the question as an opportunity to give an explanation – I don't know what I said. But I now think that I was probably seeking to reassure her and lessen her guilt. Purgatory is an in-between space, a waiting space, where the individual awaits a decision in relation to their soul's future destiny. Amy seeks an understanding of purgatory at a time when she is required to wait in the hospital until the hospital authorities decide on her future home, and this is a relevant consideration in relation to her question. It appears that Amy has resolved the question of guilt and redemption and presents herself as virtuous, her anger being righteous, she is sure of going to heaven. But there is some doubt in relation to her guilt in this material, for example, the patient who is angry with Amy thinks that Amy should be given 'beetles' for breakfast.

Thirteenth Session

Amy spoke about a nurse called 'Bullet' who seemed to be off work because of sickness. She asked if this nurse was going to return to work. Amy said that when she dies, she wants to die in her sleep. As she spoke, she was making marks with a white crayon on white paper. She also used the white crayon on brown paper but did not give up on trying to mark on the white paper. Eventually she chose to abandon the white crayon in favour of the pink. She talked of hospital staff 'doing an EEP to my head'. I told her that I thought she meant EEG – used to diagnose epilepsy. She didn't think that there was much wrong with her head although she knew that she was 'a bit slow'. It emerged that she was angry about it as 'they didn't give me anything – no cup of tea'. I connected it to here – the Art Therapy – not having tea in the beginning. She repeated that she knew she was slow but she thought that people took advantage of her. I agreed that they probably did. She drew a box. She then spoke about a man murdering his son, on TV, and this made her feel sad. Inside the box were handkerchiefs and tools – these were not drawn. She then asked did I remember her middle name. I confessed that I had forgotten – she then said that she too had forgotten mine.

Amy is thinking about sickness and death. The white crayon and its invisibility implies the presence of something that cannot be seen, found, or represented in a visible form. This use of the white crayon is followed by her account of investigations of her head, investigations searching for something that may be the cause of being a 'bit slow'. Thinking of the white crayon in relation to the pink, the white would indicate sickness and death. In the previous session we had a man who was a 'poisoner' in this session it is a man who murders his son. The sadness could link to her younger ideal brother who died. Handkerchiefs and tools are an odd mixture. The exchange around middle names suggests a desire for a more intimate connection with me. I don't remember Amy telling me her middle name. Forgetfulness in this respect may well express a wish on my part to maintain a professional distance.

Fourteenth Session

She talked of a nurse 'wanting to control her mind'. She draws, 'lines- they're lines aren't they?'. This was followed by 'four rings, circles' and 'five lines'. She then told me about 'ugly men' trying to pick her up in a car and 'a patient being raped'. The men pushed her, the patient, out of the car and 'The bastard wiped his dirty penis on a bit of newspaper'. Then she quickly moved on to her mother who 'gave her snuff when she was a few days old and this affected her brain'. Her dad told her this. Her brother died of pneumonia, and she remembered him having TB and dying. Amy then talked about going to hostels. 'They look after you in the hostels – don't they?' she asked. I suggested she was worried about being neglected – that bad things could happen to her, and she was wondering if I would be reliable? Amy then described her drawing as 'scribble like a low grade or a child' the circles, she explained, were 'gone over too much'. I said to her that she was hard on herself.

There was a lot of tragedy, trauma and pain in her material in this session. The story of the rape, with its graphic detail, did disturb me. I became anxious about my competence and Amy's fragility. I felt sure the 'patient' was her. I was very reluctant to ask questions as I didn't want to be suggestive in relation to answers. She moved on quickly from the topic and I did think that she would return to this subject, when she felt strong enough to explore it further. But my thinking was, also, I now feel, prompted by my wish to avoid difficulties.

*It is the staff from the hospital who are seeking to control her **mind** but it is her mother who is responsible for her **brain** and she again remembers the death of her younger brother. The snuff feels like an assault and maybe some murderous intent. There is the important issue of who cares for her, now and in the future. Being like a 'low grade or a child' indicates not only an awareness of vulnerability but also of having a memory of having suffered from abusive experiences that come with being vulnerable, and I can now see that I wanted to acknowledge the pain that accompanies this insight, and/or offer something that might alleviate the raw feeling, which, like the circles, is 'gone over too much'. But my responses were 'low grade'.*

Fifteenth Session

She came late and talked of 'Fat Dennis' who undressed her, another patient who robbed her, and another who borrowed money and didn't pay her back. She did not wish to use the materials today. However, she agreed to play squiggles. The first squiggle looked like a fish, then became a leg and an Easter egg with a ribbon. The second squiggle a flag on the flag pole. She then told me of a story of a Policeman who murdered three women. He was a family man and he gave them all tea first. She agreed that some men were dangerous but she said 'Not you, you're alright – you wouldn't do anything like that – I hope'. The Policeman in the story puts a baby into a home, and this reminded her of going into a home which she did not like. I asked if her father was a dangerous man. 'Yes he was' she said and he 'dug his nails into my hand'. When she was skipping, she fell and her father told her that she would be crippled for the rest of her life. She wanted to know if I had a better childhood, was hers 'bad or usual'. 'Families are like that' she concluded, 'I couldn't be angry with them (parents) now they're both dead'. I was going on holiday again (Summer holiday), and we would not be able to meet. She knew that she could go to the Victoria centre and do drawing, etc., with G. who was an art instructor, while I was away but she said, 'I won't will I it's not the same'.

Dennis's action seemed to be like the rape and nobody appears to be trustworthy – not other patients or the policeman, who was 'a family man', who gave tea but murders, and puts the baby into a home. We had previous accounts of a father murdering his son, and this naturally lead me to think about Amy's father, a father whom Amy presents as cruel. He appears to be as bad as her neglectful and murderous mother. But, as Amy points out, 'families are like that'. How bad was her childhood compared to others – that is what Amy wants to know. As her parents are now both dead she feels that she could no longer be angry with them, but is this the case? Importantly she lets me know that she hopes I can be trusted and that I will be missed during the Summer holiday.

Sixteenth Session

Amy said that she was being punished for being too slow. She was glad that her mother and father were dead (she laughed briefly). Her parents would not allow her to have bed socks and a hot water bottle at night. She then talked about Dennis mentioned in the previous session – he was 'another boyfriend' and again she related that he was undressing her. With a crayon she produced some red marks on the paper which she had placed down on the table. She told me that she had an 'Egyptian bag' which was thrown away by her brother. This bag had belonged to her mother, and it was important to Amy. I suggested that it might have been a way of remembering mother. Amy said that the bag meant that she would one day be back home. This was her hope. Her brother replaced it 'but it's not the same is it?' she said. Next she added some red paint to the red crayon marks. She thought about the result of her work, was it 'a dog, or is it a rabbit, or a male rabbit, a hare?' She next made some circular marks which she described as 'strokes'.

Amy asked a lot of questions about me in this session, so much so that I found myself stressing that the sessions were for her to explore things that were important to her. But maybe that was precisely what she was doing! 'I know you're staff aren't you' she said.

The Egyptian bag cannot be replaced, and invested in it was the hope of returning home, the hope of moving out of the hospital into a hostel is not the same. The uncertain animal she was attempting to identify through her drawing was, I now feel, a way of thinking about men, and about the therapist, this represents a contrast, in relation to the significantly female bag, which implies an identification with her mother. Her final statement indicates that she is fully aware of our differences, which includes the power that I exercise in the relationship, a power which is supported by the patriarchal institutional context. However, in knowing that I am staff, and that some questions are not answered, she knows that what I can offer is limited.

Seventeenth Session

In this session, she was not able to find a place for her handbag and the contents spilled out over the floor. She said how she was fed up with the noises on her ward, and that there were two people dying on the sick ward. She was drawing a house and asked when would she be going to a hostel. She said that she wanted to 'blow up the hospital'. 'You don't blame me do you?' she added.

There is no place for her bag, since in the hospital there is little space for hope. The spilled contents of the bag I felt signified an experience of multiple losses and in drawing a house Amy expresses her longing for a new start, in a different environment, where she is not disturbed by noises and people dying. Blowing up the hospital would certainly change things.

Eighteenth Session

Amy had missed two sessions because she had been in the sick ward. Her leg had swollen and she reminded me that she had Oedema. She spoke about not going to work with the art instructor anymore and asked 'Did I need to?' I agreed that she did not need to go. She spoke again about her slowness and 'Bullet' who called her a 'witch'. Then Amy referred to her male friends saying that she was allowing Dennis and Barry to do things to her. She had produced some black marks with a crayon which she described as 'different to each other' Her brother, she says, tells her she is 'too slow' – said with some emphasis on the 'too slow'. She asked me to speak to the art instructor and the ward so that they should know that she did not need to attend the instructor's classes, and I agreed to do this.

The art instructor provided a space for residents who wished to use art materials on a recreational basis. She is not well but she is reminded of her slowness, which does trouble her. This slow 'witch' appears passive in relation to her male friends. The slowness could be the difficulty of working things out for herself, for example in terms of the meaning of the black marks which are differentiated. Perhaps they represent her male friends, the art instructor, myself and her brother. I think dependency is fostered by the hospital staff who are insistent on making decisions for her, and haven't I just done this? Maybe this is what she wants to escape from.

Nineteenth Session

Amy talked about the art instructor again. 'I don't go to G. because I go to you' she said and added 'G is stricter than you – you have to do some work', but he does give her 'lots of tea and biscuits'. She began painting a tree and stripes. Then told me how Barry was told off for 'peeing down trousers' by the ward staff. They said to him (?) 'You can go now'. I suggested to her that she was not being listened to and not given enough time. 'That's right they don't give me enough time – I do feel that'.

She is still deciding on the difference between myself and the art instructor. The art instructor requires her to 'work' but he feeds her. The question mark I inserted into the notes at the time highlights the difficulty in knowing whether it was really Barry she was talking about or herself who was summarily dismissed. Some staff are 'strict' that's for sure.

Twentieth Session

As she did not seem to know what to do in relation to the materials I suggested, she used coloured paper. 'You're bossing me' she said. She reminded me that she liked 'purple' because 'it is the colour my mother doesn't like'. Then we spoke about holidays, I was going on holiday and so was she. At the very end of the session, she says, 'Oh... I didn't tell you Barry and me are going to a hostel in E... will you come and see me there?'

In this session, I became the strict one. Being 'bossy' is robbing her of some autonomy, of making a choice. Amy was reminding me of her conflictual relationship around 'purple' (or 'mauve') with her mother. It is related to the larger theme – the necessity of achieving independence. There is some hopeful news at the end of the session, and leaving it until the last is another way of maintaining autonomy.

Twenty-First Session

Amy arrived early and I asked her to wait as I was talking to a member of staff in the office. She then went to the toilet. When she came in, she talked about the staff throwing her out of the ward because of a meeting, and they told her to hurry saying 'if you don't join the table in 10 mins the food will be taken away'. She was drawing a house and said, 'Somebody is dying in a hostel – they're all different aren't they – the hostels'.

Being asked to wait was difficult; I needed to hurry, as she was in danger of losing something. She reminds me that you could die in a hostel and the fact that they were all different suggests that there might be bad hostels and good hostels. There is a sense here too that there is not much time left in her life.

Twenty-Second Session

She began a drawing with a semi-circular mark at the top of the paper. Gradually a figure emerged. She wanted to know if 'sleeping together' in a room with Barry was alright in a hostel. She said that the figure 'could be me'. She said how she was hungry 'You don't get enough to eat here – well you do get enough, you can have a second helping if you want'.

What would the arrangements be in the hostel and would it be what she wanted? Being hungry reminds me of the previous session and the need to hurry to get to the table. Does she get enough 'here' in the Art Therapy? Do I answer her questions and alleviate her anxieties?

Twenty-Third Session

Amy was standing very close to me today and she was reading a label on a dried milk tin, used as a jar for brushes, 'is this for babies?' she asked. There was some kind of incident with Bullet but it was hard to get a clear picture of it except Bullet broke her necklace. 'I called her a bastard – wouldn't you – she just broke it on my neck out of spite'. She was rolling plasticine as she told me this.

We have a clear reference to babies and feeding. Is the Art Therapy for babies? 'Bullet' is clearly a bad mother.

Twenty-Fourth Session

Amy was accompanied by 'Dirty Dennis' and she asked me if I could supply Dennis with a 'proper pen'. I gave her a pen which Amy then gave to Dennis who departed. She then talked of Dennis being dirty, undressing her. She was drawing a house. When she had finished the house I commented that it was 'standing alone on an empty sheet'. She did not respond verbally to my comment, but instead added curtains to the windows of the house.

Having a more fulfilling relationship with 'Dirty Dennis' is required. My comment on the house 'standing alone on an empty sheet' suggests that I was sensitive to some transmitted affect that was related to the loneliness of her situation. Adding curtains to the windows of the house makes the interior more private, or, we could say it was a matter of dressing the house, and this action undoes Dennis's undressing of her.

Twenty-Fifth Session

I visited Amy in the sick ward. She wanted Barry to visit but 'he wouldn't come in' she said. She thought that he was 'silly – frightened of staff'. I said that I could try and help. She said that she had some 'stiffness in her shoulder – arthritis as she was getting old' She asked if she would be able to come next week to Art Therapy and I reassured her that I would be 'there', in the studio.

I do not seem to have remembered much of what was exchanged between us in the sick ward – this note is very brief. My thinking at the time, I remember, was directed towards practical help, encouraging the nurses to facilitate a visit by Barry.

Twenty-Sixth Session

Amy was reluctant to enter into the studio space and instead sat in the toilet nearest the door. I said to her 'It was very difficult to come into the room today'. 'Yes well it is – well it is and it isn't – it's difficult and it isn't' she said. She asked 'Did I see anyone else when she didn't come' – meaning when in the sick-ward. She also commented that you could stay all morning if you went to see G the art instructor.

It appears that Amy feels she has missed out, because of her sickness, and there is a suggestion that I could have offered her more. Was I already transferring my attention, and affection, on to others?

Twenty-Seventh Session

Amy came late and she talked about a film of a 'mother murdering her daughter'. She then began to talk of dangerous men and a patient being stripped and cast into a ditch. I asked her if she felt that was what I might do. She responded, 'No you're not that sort of person'.

She was standing very close to me again, and she drew a 'high chair' to which she added 'a baby' (Figure 6). She commented that she used to sit in the high chair 'when I was a baby'. I asked her if she sometimes felt like a baby. She responded by saying 'Yes when I talk silly'. She then talked about babies being abandoned. She recollected that one day she lost her mother, after she came out of a shop, and she finished up in a police station. Her mother came to collect her and Amy said

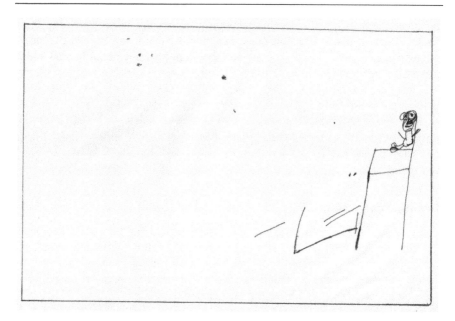

Figure 6 Baby in high chair. Original, crayon and pencil on pale red paper – A3. Tracing by the author.

to her mother, 'You're not my real mother only my step-mother'. This made her mother angry, she reported.

This was an important session. We have had a mother who murders and a mother who abandons her babies. Amy abandons her mother when she asserts, in the presence of the policeman, 'you're not my real mother'. Abandonment, and abuse, refer to traumatic past experience, and my guess is that she was that patient who was stripped and cast into the ditch. I should have linked this to her conversation about rape in Session 14 rather than asking the question about trust. I seem to be still avoiding the exploration of some material.

The baby on the high chair is very much alone. It is a small vulnerable figure who opens her arms. The features on the face, the eyes, nose and mouth, may have been 'gone over too much' as Amy has said when drawing previously (Session 14), but they add weight to the idea, that this is a baby that is pleading for a response. The lines, or 'strokes' (see Session 16), that move across the paper, begin to form a rectangle, perhaps one of her boxes, but this part of the drawing ends in a white line, near the centre, a white line which is clearly visible this time, on the red paper.

Twenty-Eighth Session

Amy drew on two sheets at once, saying, 'lines, strokes I suppose, just strokes really'. She thought of 'Dumbo and Bambi' and this made her feel sad. The 'crosses', she had drawn, 'were kisses'. I asked if she was sad when her mother left her. She said, 'My mother's dead – I didn't cry when she died – I know I should have but I didn't – I was sad when my father died'.

The idea of lines as 'strokes' returns. 'Dumbo and Bambi' suggests both intellectual disability and childhood. Amy is quite clear about her feelings in relation to her mother and her father. Who were the 'kisses' for?

Twenty-Ninth Session

She told me that her brother had a 'devil inside him' when he tore up the card given to him by her mother. She told me that she felt good getting angry with her mother 'now she's gone'. I asked her if she had a 'devil' inside her. 'Well yes but there again – don't you?' She was manipulating some plasticine between her fingers when she spoke. She said she had made 'A little ball'.

We all have a 'little devil' inside us – and this should be understood in contrast to the innocent image of childhood, the innocence of 'Bambi' and 'Dumbo'. Hatred would probably be the right word for the feeling condensed into that 'little ball'.

Thirtieth Session

Prior to this meeting, I cancelled a session at short notice to attend a meeting. Amy began the session by saying 'There was a murder in Leytonstone where you live' followed by 'Well yes I did feel like murdering you – yes I did feel like it'. She produced a drawing of 'Dr Jekyll and Mr Hyde'. He was good some of the time and bad at other times she told me; 'He grew mad – this was a madhouse B... hospital'. Amy then expressed regrets about leaving hostels, because she behaved badly. I asked if she thought she was like Dr Jeckyl. 'I suppose I am, this is a mad house – he destroyed himself, he died in the end'. She emphasised that the drawing was the 'monster part of Dr Jekyl'. In relation to the strokes on the paper, she said 'I don't mean a stroke like when you have a stroke'. Then she talked about her mother having a stroke. Her mother could not speak and was unable to say her brother's name. 'Where were you last week?' she asked. Then she said that her uncle was paralyzed by a stroke, down one-side, she liked her uncle (Figure 7).

I cannot now recollect what meeting it was that I felt it was important to attend, but I failed to communicate with Amy in person and offer an alternative time, instead, I left a message with the ward staff. There is more than a little irony to this given that Amy had been exploring her abandonment and unmet need. She had also suggested that I was not immune from hate or murderous feeling, that I also 'had a devil inside' (previous session), and certainly there was some hate, here in the countertransference, that was evidently at work, murderous feeling aroused in me as a protest against that demand, felt as excessive, for love and compassion, consideration and concern. Murderous feeling is met with murderous feeling, and Dr Jekyll and Mr Hyde supply just the right image to explore her thinking. This was the first time that she had mentioned going to a hostel previously, about which she had regrets. The 'monster part', Mr Hyde, 'destroyed himself' and Dr Jekyll, in the

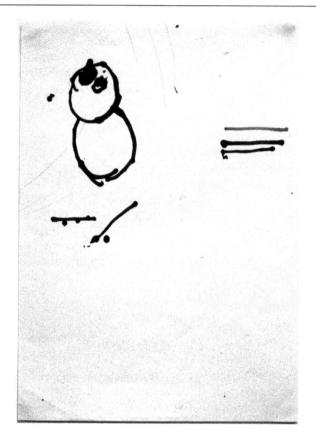

Figure 7 Figure and strokes. A4 paper and felt tip pen, some pencil.

end, and Amy regrets her mad/bad feelings. The 'strokes' do refer to her mother, and her phantasy seems to be that she is responsible for the stroke that kills, or the stroke that affects her likeable uncle (the therapist). The phrase 'down one-side' reminds me of the Spina-Bifida.

This is Dr Jekyll, or more precisely 'the monster part', Mr Hyde. He appears to be looking upwards, and if we compare this figure to the first figure that Amy drew, then we can see that this figure is very much closer to the baby on the high chair (Session 27), a figure associated with abandonment. If the lines, or strokes, are to be identified with the marks to the right of the figure and underneath the figure, then they also suggest unattached limbs, and the figure then becomes a figure falling into pieces. There are some feint pencil lines that cross the figure or descend from above, and the left edge of the paper, these could also be thought of as strokes – we are not sure. In relation to Dr Jeckyll and Mr Hyde, it is important that we recognise a reference to the therapist as well as Amy herself. The therapist shares the same murderous feelings that members of staff are capable of exhibiting when relating to residents in the hospital, and it is important for Amy to establish this fact.

Thirty-First Session

Amy arrived early asking which toilet should she use – the handicapped one or the non-handicapped one. I waited in the studio space. After some time in the toilet, she talked to Barry who was waiting outside the door. She asked me if Barry could wait inside and I said 'No'. She then tells me he has a bad cold and shouldn't be outside 'he should be on the ward'. I said to her that Barry isn't my responsibility and went on to suggest that she is worried about him not looking after himself. She said, 'I told him to stay where its warm – he wants to go to the canteen with me'. After some reflection, she said, 'Yes he can' look after himself. During this exchange, she kept her coat and hat on and remained standing. 'I told him you'd say no'. I suggested, 'You're thinking maybe I'm hard on him, punishing him'. Her colour changes, and she is clearly embarrassed, 'Yes punishing him, cruel, but he doesn't work here does he'. 'No', I say, 'this space is for you'.

Amy then decides to use the crayons, then she reads the labels on the crayon box, out loud. I then suggested to her that she was demonstrating her reading skills. She then told me that somebody has died, but she is not able to go to the funeral because she wants to go shopping.

She abandoned the crayons and as she talked she divided clay into pieces, each separate piece was in turn divided into two. One piece was briefly modelled. 'It's not a dog and it's not a cat', She said. Amy then asked if I had a TV. I said 'only a wireless'. 'Is it an English wireless?' she asked. She pointed out that Barry is still outside – he could be heard coughing. She tells me of a murder on TV. The story was not immediately apparent in the telling but the gist of it was that a woman kills her lover or husband, or a man, because he killed her lover/husband. I related it to Barry being outside and put it to her that she felt that I was killing her lover, or husband, and that she wanted to kill me. 'Yes I do – I do feel that – I wouldn't really because I'd end up in gaol wouldn't I – I expect you want to kill your wife sometimes but you wouldn't would you?' 'No', I say, but I agreed that she was right 'I can have the same feelings'.

The clay is cut into more pieces, she says, 'Not a dog or a cat or any animal it's five pieces'. After this, she cut another piece into two. I point out the cutting in two and refer back to Dr Jekyl and Mr Hyde of the previous week and I suggest that maybe she feels divided in two. 'You haven't got a TV', she says. 'did you read the book will you get a TV?'. I said, 'Maybe you feel I should get a TV to get up to date, to understand you better'. She responded, 'You're old fashioned – you might understand me better if you had a TV'.

It is Barry who is abandoned now, and my inflexibility and cruelty are high-lighted as I am determined to maintain the boundaries or the 'rules' of my Art Therapy practice. Barry's appearance in this session enables Amy to emphasise her concern for others, but also my cruelty, as a member of staff. Amy is also demonstrating that she is not 'handicapped', she can look after herself, as can Barry, and she is capable of reading, for instance. Nevertheless, there is some uncertainty about her status, as she wants to hear from me which is the right toilet for her.

Not going to the funeral but going shopping instead is difficult to make sense of, but if the 'somebody' who died was a person with a learning disability, not going could be a way of showing that the funerals of people with learning disabilities are not important. I am also thinking that this was an oblique comment on my cancelling the session, and maybe Amy is wondering if I would go to her funeral. How important is the Art Therapy for me, how important is it that I continue to meet Amy on a regular weekly basis, even when the sessions become funereal? How important was the event that kept me away?

Amy learnt that I was without a TV, I only possessed a wireless. She does feel that I am killing Barry and she would like to kill me but the important thing here again is to establish my murderous feelings. My handicap is being old-fashioned and thereby not fully understanding her, and she would have liked to have seen more care and concern on my part.

Thirty-Second Session

She arrived 40 minutes late and said that she had been on the ward with Barry. She said that her night dress was stolen by the staff. She wanted to know if I was angry with her. I asked her what she thought. 'Yes you are a little – I think you are, will you give my place to someone else?' She began drawing some 'lines – strokes – three lines – rubbish really'. After a further 'three strokes' she drew a 'box'. She had some money in her hand which she almost left behind. Then after noticing this, she gave more reports about the stolen night dress. I asked her if she thought I was stealing from her – drawings and other things. 'No you're not – well you could be couldn't you – what did you do with the drawings?' – She asked.

Amy wants to know exactly what my feelings are in relation to her. She wants to know about my inclinations or motivations. Will I simply give her place to someone else, if she comes late? The strokes may need to be contained in the box. Was the money a bribe or was I meant to steal it? Amy knows that I keep her drawings in a folder and that she has access to this folder.

Thirty-Third Session

She arrived late and went into the toilet. In the studio, she wanted to remove her coat and is unable or unwilling to begin. After blowing her nose, she could not decide whether or not to place the tissues in the bin, in fact she was showing me her snot, pushing it under my face, in an aggressive way as if threatening to smear it over me. She talked about Bullet telling her off. I said that I felt she wanted me to tell her off. She then reported men shouting at her 'have you got your knickers on to-day', they were calling her a 'mental defective'. She also reported that a nurse did not believe that she had Spina Bifida. Amy follows her angry expressions of frustration quietly, but desperately, she asks 'Am I mental?' She draws a circle saying that could be 'an apple or an orange', and she adds a table and decides that it is an 'orange on a table'. She talked again about being 'mental' and she said that she should have had 'special education' but because her mother was 'carrying another baby it was not possible'.

She then told me that her brother died but 'dad said had he lived he would have died in the war'. She didn't blame her brother 'It wasn't his fault' it was her 'mother really – but you can't blame her because she is in heaven now'. Orange was her mother's favourite colour and this reminded her of her auntie who died in hospital. She had a stroke and 'had to stay in the hospital until she died' she reported. I asked her if she thought that she, herself, 'might die in the hospital'. 'Don't be like that – so morbid – do you want me to die – do you want to get rid of me?' It is time to go and she then talks about somebody being strict. I said, 'I am going to be strict now as it is the end of the session'.

In this session and the previous session her depression or melancholia was very much in evidence through her lack of care in relation to her appearance, and the snot reminded me of Barry and my 'cruelty' (see Session 31). Amy wants me to identify or name her mental state in some way. Is it imagined that I simply think that she is a 'mental defective' and deserves to be abused and insulted? I was struggling with her question about her mental state, just as she was struggling to differentiate the apple from the orange. I did think that she was right, she should have had the 'special education' and the opportunity that it might have provided for her. However, I felt that any comment on this loss would only increase the pain that she experiences when she reflects on her past. It was not the younger brother, an ideal figure for Amy, who was to blame. In this account of her ideal younger brother, the child that her mother was carrying, he appears as a replacement for Amy, in terms of her mother's care. It is, as we might expect, her mother who is to blame for her current situation, where Amy faces a death like her Auntie in hospital. But she does want to forgive her mother in this session. Orange is her mother's favourite colour and her mother is blameless and in heaven now. Towards the end of the session, I was encouraging Amy to think what may have been very difficult for her to think at that moment, and when the ending of the session arrived, it ended abruptly, through the exercise of **my** *strictness. The important question for Amy is 'do I want to get rid of her', like her mother.*

Thirty-Fourth Session

Amy reported that Bullet had been 'forcing food down her' making her 'eat faster'. This was 'because of the cleaners – it's alright for them, they go home in the afternoon, but this is my home and it's my lunch'. She said that she had lost a letter from her brother because she was careless, and she thought that a resident, 'M...' had stolen it. Amy insisted that she did want to read the letter and told me that replying to the letter took a long time, it was 'difficult to write letters in the hospital'. She then told me that the social worker had told her that she would have to stay another year in the hospital. Amy said she wanted to 'get out of this madhouse – it was horrible here'. She didn't want to end her days here. She then returned to the subject of Bullet forcing food down her and 'M...' stealing from her. I suggested that she might feel that 'I was forcing food down her – my thoughts – and also stealing her secrets'. 'Don't be silly' she responded, 'Not you, I don't mean you'. 'OK' I said, 'These are real experiences and you have a horrible time in the hospital – but you do seem to be saying that I force my thoughts on you and steal your secrets – you tell me things'. After this she said 'You don't know another person's thought' however she did agree that I did 'steal secrets'. Amy continued to emphasise how horrible life in the hospital was, how especially horrible Bullet was – 'She's got a brick swinging in her heart'. Amy then tried drawing Bullet – 'She's got some good faults – this is the top of her head'. Amy was wanting to change the colour, away from black but she had difficulty in choosing another colour. She chose black again and then moved on to blue. She emphasised again how horrible the hospital was and asked 'What about your week-end?' I suggest that she is saying 'it's alright for you – you don't live here' (something she has said before) 'you don't know what is like'. She had some difficulty in leaving at the end of the session and her drawing remained unfinished. Later she came back to look for her letter which she had lost again.

Amy's report about eating reminded me of my comment at the end of the previous session and the manner in which the session ended, abruptly with my 'strictness'. Thoughts about death take quite a bit of digesting and the social worker has just told her that she may now have to spend another year in the hospital, something else unpalatable and impossible to digest.

It is difficult to read and write letters in the hospital, it takes time to do this and the hospital being a 'horrible' place does not allow enough time. If things are forced down her, this also applies to my interpretations and, quite rightly, Amy observes that I do not 'know another person's thoughts'. Nevertheless, she is willing to acknowledge that I could be seen to be one who is 'stealing secrets'. In describing 'Bullet' I was struck by her vivid use of metaphor. 'Bullet', I think, represents all members of staff, in their strictness, and cruelty, and this includes the therapist. If I am to be a 'Bullet' does it also mean that I have some 'good faults' which are maybe related to the 'top of my head', the place from which my thoughts and words seemingly originate?

The colour for 'Bullet' has to be black and blue (which suggests bruising to me now), and her question about the week-end emphasises the fact that it is she, Amy, who lives in the horrible hospital and experiences the resulting feeling that emerges from her situation. The final search for the letter at the end of the session now suggests to me that Amy was trying to recover some message, it may have come from her mother, or her brother, but it may be the message she has received from my comments, and having access to the message would enable her to think about the issues that were existentially important to her, despite the pain that comes with it.

Thirty-Fifth Session

Amy was very late arriving just ten minutes before the end of the session time. She told me again that the hospital was horrible, 'it's alright for you – you're an outsider'. I say, 'you're punishing me because I don't live here – in the hospital – I don't have to put up with it all – it's easy for me – you're angry with me for being an outsider'. Amy responded, 'Yes that's right' and laughed 'you don't know what it is like'.

I was being punished by her lateness, but we might also ask why is Amy being punished in the 'horrible hospital'. The important thing from Amy's perspective is that I should feel, that is, be aware of the level of her depression or melancholia, because I do not experience 'what it is like'.

Thirty-Sixth Session

She came late again and told me that another patient who had the same Christian name as her 'a low-grade' fell down a manhole and hit her head. 'She should be retired from work' adding that she was now 62. I said, 'Maybe you're feeling that you should be retired from here – perhaps coming here hurts your head'. She agreed 'Yes you could say that – it does hurt my head coming here'. Then Amy asked, 'Do you want me to stop coming?'. I simply replied 'No'. She began drawing, 'a red stroke – line in red – a red stroke or line'. The girl who fell down the manhole, Amy suggested, 'threw herself down on purpose – it was 'suicide''. She said she wouldn't do it herself, 'it was silly'. I said, 'you feel very depressed'. Amy responded, 'Yes I am you would be'.

Amy imagines herself as being that 'low grade' who fell down the 'manhole'. Amy now needs to be retired. If her head is now hurting because of Art Therapy was it a kind of suicide to volunteer herself for this kind of 'work'? Her depression is such that it does lead her toward suicidal thoughts.

Thirty-Seventh Session

This session was also brief due to Amy arriving late. She produced some drawings which she described as 'Scribble, silly, not any good, really just a line'. She talked about her money being stolen and an 'equaliser man with a beard being thrown down the stairs'.

As Amy became more depressed she lost her confidence in her abilities. What she had has been stolen, and that man with a beard needs to be punished. I do have a beard.

Thirty-Eighth Session

Late arriving Amy began by talking about a radio given to Barry, 'he messes it up it's no good giving him anything'. She said that she had tried to tell staff, and referring to a nurse, 'I have to listen to her point of view but she doesn't listen to mine'. She repeated, 'it's serious – the radio will be messed up'. I linked the 'messed up' to coming late, 'messing up the Art Therapy sessions'. Amy answered that she could look after things, but Barry didn't listen. Then she talked about Dennis wanting her to rub his cock. She complained that she went to the toilet 'to have a shit and he comes in and wants me to rub his cock – filthy'. She was going to see him 'but not let him do anything dirty'.

This material seemed to require further interpretation but I did not go beyond the being late theme. Somebody is not listening and it's likely to be me, that is, a member of staff, as well as Amy herself. Having to rub Dennis's 'cock' etc., suggests the idea that she is expected to admire my interpretations, or thinking, when all she wants is to evacuate. The radio reminds me of the earlier discussion about radio and TV (Session 31) and messing up the radio seems to suggest a 'messing up' of mind. The feeling is that we are both messing up each other's mind, with our differing 'point[s] of view'.

Thirty-Ninth Session

Amy continued to talk about Dennis and how he made her strip in the caravan and sprayed her with some spray in a can. She wasn't sure what it was but she thought it was dirty. He had thrown her out of the caravan the previous night as she had been going back to the caravan to look for a bra. Dennis, she suggested, was dirty, but she did get something from him – a cup of tea or a cigarette. She began drawing a house using a very tatty piece of paper. 'Barry' she told me 'goes on about the Easter Parade' all the time. I suggested to her that perhaps she wants a 'normal boyfriend – one who isn't perverse like Dennis and one who isn't silly like Barry'. Amy said that she did have a third boyfriend 'Jim with a stick'. She did agree, in relation to Dennis, 'that's right he is perverse' and added 'you're not like him'. She thought Barry 'normal'. The house she was drawing was a 'thatched house' (Figure 8). She told me that 'someone had just gone to a bungalow with their boyfriend' and she would like to go to a hostel with Barry.

There was an old caravan, on an empty stretch of meadow at the back of the hospital which patients used as a meeting place, away from the gaze of the staff. Some staff knew this existed and were happy to leave things as they were, other staff wanted the caravan removed and seemed more interested in restricting private contact between residents. What Amy appears to be looking for is some kind of ordinary, normal, relationship. She is still hoping for a new start.

Amy's choice of a grey and grubby piece of paper with a torn edge mirrored her feelings about the dirty stuff that Dennis had sprayed her with. Just as the caravan, where the spraying took place, is very close to the hospital boundary this image of the hoped-for 'thatched house' is placed near to the torn edge of the paper. It's odd that Amy described it as 'thatched' as it appears to have tiles – the idea of a 'thatched' house suggests an ideal country cottage. A door has been placed between the windows on the ground floor of the house. The door appears to have a lock or a letter box in the centre of it. However, it is possible to interpret the door as another window. Although the house is distant there is a path to the house. The path does not go the door between the windows but goes to the side of the house, by making an abrupt turn. We are unable to view the side of the house. If Amy follows the path – will she find a door at the side?

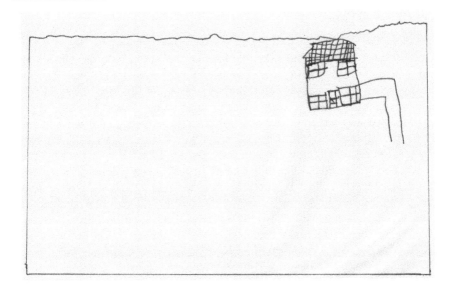

Figure 8 Thatched house and path. Original, pencil on grey A3 paper. Tracing by the author. The outer line denotes the edge of the paper which was torn along the top edge.

Fortieth Session

She told me that three people had 'just died' and 'there were funerals'. She then asked 'if you go unconscious do you come round – can you come round?'. Amy told me that she had been watching the film 'the ten commandments' and the cleaner changed the channels. She was annoyed as she wanted to watch it. Her mother had told her to watch this film, if she ever got the chance – 'before you die'. Amy said she was 'very annoyed'. I tried to connect the religious element in the film to her thoughts about death but Amy did not appear to understand my thinking. She commented, in relation to her drawing, 'I haven't done much work – mauve – lines four lines'.

Amy had experienced a loss of consciousness in the sick ward (see Session 25) so it would be reasonable for her to have fears in relation to this way of dying. She was angry about a situation where she was gaining some understanding by watching a film, and the channels were abruptly changed. This could relate to her experiences in the sick ward. But her mother's communication was clearly important to her, and has stayed with her. 'The ten commandments' is likely to carry an ethical and religious message, and there was some urgency in Amy's desire to retrieve this content. 'Mauve' is Amy's colour, and the colour that her mother does not like (Session 1). The 'four lines' could be renamed as four 'strokes'. This would imply that the cleaner was not the real target of her anger. If it is mother it is because the message from her cannot be easily retrieved and the meaning deciphered.

Forty-First Session

Amy came late and I wanted to get a clearer understanding of the lateness and I asked her what made her late. She told me that she had been to the canteen and 'had some coffee and toast in there'. I suggested that maybe it was better than here. She responded, 'No you always see things from your point of view'. Then she went on to tell me that she was given 'cold tea in the morning – it was an insult'. I then suggested that she feels empty inside before coming here. 'Yes I do' and Amy then told me that a nurse 'nearly drowned her in the bath' and 'nurses hit another patient' and 'you can't do anything because nobody saw it – I did but nobody else'. Then she repeated 'you wouldn't like to live here'. Amy then began drawing 'a box with stripes' and it had 'lid which is open'. I returned to the insult idea and feeling empty and I asked if it was difficult to come here 'because I made you think about bits of yourself you don't like to think about'. 'What was that?' she asked 'bits of myself – I've never thought of it like that before – it could be I suppose'. 'The box was open' I said, 'What's going to come out of the box?' 'You are', she said laughing.

*It's important that I listen to **her** point of view, she is insulted, nearly drowned and has to witness abuse, for which there is no remedy. Although I now think that the 'bits of yourself' idea was not particularly useful, Amy seemed able to respond to it. I was probably boxed in with my 'psychotherapeutic' theory and frame, which was constricting my thoughts and inhibiting responses. Her humour, and laughter, was refreshing – she seemed to be suggesting that she wasn't going to put up with my rubbish. I needed to be open and honest.*

Forty-Second Session

Amy came late, and this time she blamed it on Jim. I suggested to her that she was not taking responsibility for her actions. She agreed and talked about a 'spiteful girl'. This girl goes to the dentist because of pains in her teeth but complains because the dentist only gives her 'ointment which is no good – doesn't take the tooth out'. This spiteful girl also complains about pains in her stomach and 'in her head' and 'period pains'. I suggested that this spiteful girl was really like her, she comes here, which is like going to the dentist, but 'I can't take the pains away' and I wondered if 'coming here, makes you feel worse'. Amy reassured me, 'you do help'. Then she told me that Jim was waiting for her. I observed that she kept a lot of people waiting, 'me, the nurse, Barry'. She told me that she didn't keep her brother waiting anymore and again she reminded me that I would not like it 'here in the hospital – you wouldn't like to live here'. Some people had left and she was fed up with waiting – she didn't want to stay here. She was drawing a flag and I remarked on how the two lines crossed on the flag.

Art therapy doesn't remove the pain of living in the hospital but it does help. She was fed up with waiting – for the relief that a fresh beginning, in a hostel, might bring. Maybe I felt that the lines crossing on the flag said something about her anger, and my being cross with her, demanding that she take responsibility for her lateness. Being 'spiteful' would include keeping others waiting.

Forty-Third Session

Amy came eight minutes before the end. She told me that she had to search for a 'low-grade'. I linked her lateness to the previous week and her waiting for the hostel and I suggested that this, coming late, was a way of letting me feel how bad the waiting is. Amy laughed nervously.

It is the 'low-grade' that keeps her away, maybe the 'low-grade' that fell down the manhole (Session 36). If thinking is painful and staying away is the only way to avoid this pain, coming eight minutes before the end is a way of communicating her pain. Her feelings about waiting may only be a small part of what generates the pain.

Forty-Fourth Session

Amy was only five minutes late. She said that Jim was waiting outside and she was anticipating a fight between him and Barry. She said that Jim was jealous. Then she asks about the forthcoming Whitsun holiday. She told me that she had 'sessions with Michele' and 'we talk about aids and sex'. As she spoke she drew a house and she asked 'is it alright'. We can hear Barry and Jim arguing. 'Can you hear them fighting?' she asks and seems excited by this. I asked her if she wanted this to happen – 'I did and I didn't'. I then asked if her Mother and Father ever had fights. Then I felt perhaps this was too much of a leap as she then asked aggressively if my parents ever fought. I said 'Yes, sometimes'. She then agreed that her Mother and Father did fight. She then returned to the subject of Jim's jealousy and the fight with Barry which could be heard. I asked her if she thought I might be jealous of Michele – if she wanted us to fight. She responded as she often did with this kind of question, 'I do and I don't'. Then Amy moved on to the subject of hostels reminding me of how many years she had been here and how it was hard to wait all the time – 'you wouldn't like it'. I asked, in relation to the drawing in which there were two houses nearing completion, if the house with all the different colours was the home she wanted. 'Could be', she replied and finished her drawing by adding a roof to the second house.

Jealousy seems to be the theme, and male/female relations. Amy also wants to engineer conflict; somebody or some bodies, to do the fighting for her, the fighting with the hospital and her brother, for instance, and this excites her. Michele was part of the 'resettlement team' and I was aware that she was offering Amy some counselling, and I was thinking that Amy wanted me to know that she had important relations and conversations with other members of staff. Maybe the excitement of witnessing a fight offers her some relief from the pain of waiting, and the pain of knowing how long she has been in the hospital waiting.

Forty-Fifth Session

She wanted to know if Barry was going to meet Jim again. Then she said she met a 'strange man' who was asking where the 'expression building' was. I suggested that he must have meant 'extension building' but she was sure, 'No, I think it was expression'. Amy then told me that she went to the woods with Dennis who 'stripped her naked – but he didn't have any cream come out of his cock, you know that spunk man's spunk'. She went on to say that they got lost in the woods, 'there was a garden, a maze, but we saw a gap and a way out in the end'. Then she mentioned that Barry was going to the woods 'to meet the murderers up there with guns – what was Barry going to do it was silly'. I attempted to link the story to the transference, and Amy laughed at the idea of me being like Dennis. I then tried another angle suggesting that the story was like a fairy story – 'being in the woods where there was a garden and a maze where you could get lost'. Amy then asked 'what happened in the story'. I asked what story she might be thinking about and she suggested 'Hansel and Gretel' and 'being gobbled up by a witch'. 'Dennis was good really – he didn't leave me' she said. During all this she was drawing 'strokes', one mark represented 'a bit of wood'. Dennis she told me had struck her on the neck with a bit of wood.

All three of her male friends appear in this material. Barry and Jim offer excitement through the possibility of fighting, whereas Dennis offers another kind of excitement. But the lack of 'spunk' suggests a lack of fulfilment in her sexual relations. For me at that time it reminded me of the abstinence rule in psychotherapy and this tempted me into the botched 'transference interpretation'. Dennis did provide safety, and a way out was found 'in the end' which suggests some hope is kept alive. After my intervention, it becomes the place where hungry children are trapped by a voracious and wicked witch. Dennis 'was good really', nevertheless his actions with a bit of wood did appear to be murderous. Striking on the neck implies a beheading, and the 'strokes' on the paper bring the action into mind. The 'expression' building can only be the Art Therapy department and the speech and language department which shared the same building and surely the 'strange man' at the beginning was reminding her of where to go.

Forty-Sixth Session

Amy told me that her brother visited but she didn't make him wait anymore. She made it clear that she was very angry with him. 'Do you know what he said to me, he insulted me, said I couldn't go to the hostel because I couldn't do my own washing and go to the shops and buy my own clothes – It was an insult', she said, and continued, 'Sister told me they look after you in the hostel anyway – he says I like it here in the hospital – would you like living here?' Amy informed me that her brother does not allow her to go home 'because he claims that I would wet the mattress and he'd have to hang it out of the window'. There followed a long monologue which was, like many of Amy's monologues, difficult to follow;

My mother used to allow me to go home on Wednesday afternoons. This afternoon I would be going home. I was 14 when I was sent to the hospital. My youngest brother had blond hair he was beautiful – he died of pneumonia and

TB. He was on a bus with my mum, his nose was running, a woman on the bus told my mother that she wasn't looking after him. He was neglected. My dad says it was my mum and my mum says it was my dad.

She then told me that her dad hit her 'with a belt across my bottom, and he dug his nails into me when I was sitting on his lap'. Dad 'rowed' with her mother, he 'threw the chips into the air' and called her mother 'a fat bitch'. In relation to mother, she said, 'I remember very clearly she chased me round the table with a knife, a bread knife – I ran down the stairs – I didn't get the lift – I ran away'. I asked 'were you very frightened?' 'Yes I was', she responded, but she couldn't remember why her mother was angry but she did say 'she had a hard life'. Amy said, with emphasis, that she didn't want to 'die here', she wanted to 'get to a hostel'. I then reminded her of Dr Jekyll and I said that it was not surprising that you have had murderous thoughts about killing people when all this had happened to you. She agreed and seemed to understand. We had gone over time with this monologue and Amy asked for tea but I said that it was time for us to stop.

Her brother does not allow her to visit him and he insults her. Her mother was not as cruel and did allow regular visits. Amy was angry and the long monologue that followed was suffused with feeling. Her younger brother appears as a 'beautiful' child in this monologue, an ideal image, or figure. 'His nose running' reminds me of Barry and of Amy thrusting her snot into my face (see Sessions 33 and 31). This image of the beautiful but neglected child is contrasted with the image of her sadistic father and her neglectful murderous mother. Her mother's murderous intentions, and the expression of these, frightened her. Although her mother could be excused because she had a 'hard life'.

Amy, as she understands her situation, is now in danger of dying in the hospital, but she is still hoping to go to a hostel and her capacity to reflect on her past must help in relation to her own murderous thoughts. This contrasts with the previous session which was focussed on the present and contained more in the way of phantasy. I think that I must have been trying to lessen her guilt, and her anxieties, with my more reassuring comment at the end. It was interesting for me to learn that Amy did visit her mother and I wondered when it was exactly that her mother died. This was not in the documents I was able to access. I could have, of course, asked Amy! Did I consider the question to be too painful? I did have to stop the session abruptly as we went over time.

Forty-Seventh Session

Amy came late and said that somebody in the canteen is 'spoiling for a fight'. 'You don't know what it is like in our villa – the potatoes half cooked', she said. She wanted me to know that the member of staff who tells her she is slow 'lives with her brother-in-law – is that legal?' – 'her husband hit her, some men are bad, you wouldn't do that but you didn't give me any drink last week did you?' I suggested that she was 'spoiling for a fight' and 'looking for fault – the staff tell her what to do – but they do things that are not legal' and I went on to say that I thought she came late to let me know how she felt about not getting tea. Amy said that Barry says she is slow and I point out how everybody says it. Amy then describes 'a resident who is very slow, all the time, and says she is going to do things in her time because her brother is a bastard'. I said, 'it sounds like you'. 'Yes – I am slow, my brother is a bastard, he will not let me go home, he keeps me here, he treats me badly', she replied. I then added that being, or going slow, is 'the only protest you can make. You're stuck here so you're going to make sure that you do things at your own pace'. Amy says that her brother 'does make her angry'.

Amy was hurrying to complete a drawing – 'it's not a house – nearly – it's a square really – there's a bit going off here'.

The fight between us is out in the open. The institution does not provide her with a good feed, and instead of giving her tea I offer meaningless reassurance. I think now she was telling me that she also needed more time – 'the potatoes half cooked'. But it was difficult for me to see this since I was embroiled in a conflictual relation with her around the lateness. I wanted a consistent time with a consistent boundary. Not giving tea must be illegal, if not as bad as 'hitting' her. The conversation does enable her to clarify matters in relation to her slowness. Others might see her slowness as evidence of her intellectual disabilities, but Amy uses her slowness to punish others and to assert her independence. It's her brother who makes her angry, because he could let her go home. Maybe to a place where she might properly be cared for? The square and the 'bit going off' imply another box, with a lid, for the containment of feeling.

Forty-Eighth Session

Thirty minutes late this time and stayed in the toilet for ten minutes. When coming into the studio Amy asks if she can go back to the toilet to fetch a doll and a card left behind. I'm despairing thinking that we had made progress. Amy apologises for being late and blames Barry and a staff member. She said that she had told the member of staff that he (Barry) should go to the canteen and the staff member had told her that she shouldn't interfere. We could both hear Barry and Jim outside arguing. 'Listen they're rowing', she said. I commented that we were 'rowing' in here. Amy laughs – 'I suppose we are'. She was late for breakfast but got there for tea and toast and the staff were very angry with her. I then spoke about my anger and despair, I said, 'I thought we had made progress but you are late again' and I then said that I thought she came late so that I could feel angry for her. 'Good job you're not my brother' she responded and then emphasised how she didn't like 'living here'. Amy reported that a member of staff was told off by the sister, she was 'bawling, crying' and contrasted this with how she herself didn't do this when 'someone wiped the floor with her'. I returned to the lateness and tried to emphasise that it had to be her decision in relation to coming on time but that I was aware that she was losing an opportunity. I stressed that I was available for one hour. Then I wondered if she was confused by my messages.

The spell in the toilet replicates her behaviour towards her brother, and in this way, Amy continues the fight between us. She is fighting with the staff and she is enjoying the fight between Barry and Jim. Following some honesty about my feelings, Amy points out that 'Living here' is the source of her pain, and then she asserts that she would not have given way to tears, like the abused member of staff. There is also an implication that if I were her brother it might be even more painful for me. I stressed the boundaries at the end of the session. I suppose I wanted her to make her decisions in relation to attendance in a thoughtful way, but maybe that is naïve, given the feeling she is struggling with. I wonder now what Amy might have said had I suggested that really she was telling me that she wanted more time.

Forty-Ninth Session

Forty minutes late this time. She bought with her a new cup *for her* tea. She repeated 'you would be slow if you lived here'. She did no drawing but said 'it only hurts me in the end'.

What she needs is tea in a new cup. Some special feeding perhaps. She knows she is 'messing up' like Barry and his radio (Session 38) and that she punishes herself. Or, maybe it is the drawing, and by extension thinking, that 'hurts… in the end'.

Fiftieth Session

Forty-five minutes late and Amy excused this lateness by telling me that it was 'because a patient stole her money'. 'Michelle' she said has 'finished with her – it was only for 12 weeks'. She was expecting a letter from her brother but has not received one. She wanted to know if I was angry with her for keeping me waiting.

Michele has now abandoned her and her brother has not written, what she did have has been stolen. What did it feel like to be 'finished with' after 12 weeks? Could I still be angry with her? Maybe were I to be angry with her she would know that I had some feelings for her (see Session 48).

Fifty-First Session

Thirty minutes late and Amy suggests it is 'sister's fault'. She lost her socks and tights. Then she adds, 'I suppose it is my fault really'. There was a telephone call in the canteen, 'I thought it was you but you wouldn't ring would you – you couldn't care less could you'. She was drawing a 'box' which she described as 'not much really'. She told me that she was reported for putting her hand into the swill bin, but she complained to the nursing staff as this was 'not true'. Her brother was not coming on Sunday and there was a 'deaf and dumb girl crying in her bed at night all alone', and there was 'nobody to visit her'.

Reluctantly she accepts that she is at fault but a telephone call from me would have shown her that I had feeling, that I cared for her however wretched she felt about herself. Putting her hand into the swill bin would be an indication of how desperate she can feel, but it also indicates a transgression. Perhaps she thinks that others regard her as unclean. Crying at night all alone, being without visitors, might well end in her becoming deaf and dumb, if her depression deepens.

Fifty-Second Session

She was late again because her money was stolen again. She had a card from Michelle who is now in America – but this was stolen also. 'Drives you mad here' she said. She told sister that she has bad nerves, but sister doesn't believe her. I suggested to her that maybe she (Amy) means something else. 'No I don't' she responded angrily, and I commented on how angry and depressed she is – 'Well you would be wouldn't you Robin'.

Money has gone again and an important communication is stolen. I fail to appreciate what she is trying to tell me. What does she mean by 'bad nerves'? Oddly, or perhaps not so oddly, I do now remember my mother saying she had 'bad nerves' and my not understanding at the time.

Fifty-Third Session

Amy came on time, but she spent ten minutes in the toilet at the beginning of the session. During the session, she slept, and when she woke, I said how very tiring everything was for her. She did some drawing, some 'strokes, lines and circles', which she named as 'flowers'.

She is trying to change the murderous 'strokes' the 'lines and circles', which are repetitive, into something more positive. The flowers could be a gift, a way of making a peace treaty. Everything was very tiring for both of us.

Fifty-Fourth Session

As Amy was 30 minutes late, I asked if she wanted to come. 'I do and I don't', she replied. She tells me that she is going to a hostel in January and moving to a new ward at the end of the month. She then talked about a 'little boy who was lost and who has been murdered by a man with a moustache'. Then Barry goes into the forest to look for murderers. She told me it was not safe in the woods, and she mentioned red riding hood who was eaten by a wolf. As she was speaking she was drawing with a white oil pastel on white paper, 'two lines but you can't see them' she informed me.

The little boy who was lost and murdered could be her younger brother, with whom she identifies and idealizes. She wants to ensure that she does not get lost in the woods, where she is in danger of being devoured. The white lines on the white paper re-introduce the thing that cannot be given visible form, and maybe it has ancient origins in some primitive oral aggression, emerging from some dark forest. The white lines could be regarded as 'strokes'.

Fifty-Fifth Session

Only five minutes late. There is a girl who complains of not having any money. Amy says that 'she can get it – if she goes and gets it – can't she'. Some people had left her villa and she will miss them. She wants to draw a house but is not sure whether to use a large sheet of paper or a small sheet. She decides on a large sheet and is pleased with the house as it progresses. There are further complaints about the girl and the money – she had to learn to wait, like Amy herself. Another girl moved to her villa and she should recognise Amy as she is 'an old friend'. She adds a chimney to her house. She is going to see the hostel in January and move in March and will be glad to 'get out of here'. She tells me 'the Refuge fell through', then says 'don't say that'. She adds a figure to her picture which is her when younger and when she had blonde hair. Then she described a film where a large black eagle goes around murdering people, like the little boy. I said it sounds like death. 'It is death' she says emphatically. Then she says how she has had 45 years of 'wasted life', here in the hospital. A second house was completed but the figure remained incomplete.

I wasn't sure where the girl was supposed to get the money from. Amy has seen others leave her Villa and she now has to begin to make relations with new residents. The reference to the Refuge is a reference to the earlier, failed attempt at 'resettlement' in a hostel (see Session 30). Her drawing, emphasising blond hair, brings her closer to her past and her younger brother who then appears as a 'little boy'. 'Death' is in close proximity but what is painful in this session is 'wasted life'.

Fifty-Sixth Session

Thirty minutes late. Amy asks 'will you miss me when I've gone?' She chooses 'Black, dark paper' and draws an 'apple and a ring' and asks 'shall I fill it in?'. She tells me there is 'somebody dying' and 'a funeral'. Her brother stopped coming, 'when we had a row about me going to the toilet – but it's alright now I think'. 'Pity you don't have a TV', she remarked, and then described 'The prisoner'.

> She tried to kill him at first, then he got the better of her. Tonight you can see what he did to her – I'm looking forward to that – she was forced to go into this room and work with him – that's how it started.

I related all this to the two of us and also reminded her of the man with moustache. She couldn't believe that I could be 'like the murderer'. At the end of the session, she draws 'a stroke – a line' on her paper. Finally, she asks if she would go to the lavatory in the hostel when her brother visits.

There will be an end to our relationship if she does manage to get to a hostel. The apple makes me think of Eve's gift to Adam, and the ring suggests a marriage, 'filling in' the ring would be to put her finger in the ring. The 'black dark paper', the dying and the funeral indicate that she is anticipating her own death. Things are better with her brother. But I did feel that the story from the TV brings the contention in relationships back to her experiences in Art Therapy. The TV is to remind me that I am not capable of understanding. If I am not the man with the moustache, that is a murderous man, then I am 'the prisoner' who she has tried to kill and is maybe going to do something 'to her' that she is 'looking forward to'! A bit like Dennis in that respect. Amy is still producing 'strokes'. Finally, will she continue to hate her brother, will she still need to communicate her feelings through her actions, or will things change? We know he does not want her at home because she will wet the bed (see Session 46); he comes to visit and she goes to the toilet. Is this going to the toilet a reminder of his complaint? The incontinence is a problem for Amy herself, maybe a really difficult one, given her spina-bifida, and it could be that her communications in relation to this issue have been consistently ignored. Of course, Amy does enjoy the fight with her brother, as she does with me.

Fifty-Seventh Session

Amy explained that she missed the previous week because she bought 'a low grade' tea in the canteen. She told me that 'Dirty Dennis' wanted her to push her finger into his bottom. She liked and didn't like doing it. I suggested to her that she wanted me to know how dirty she could be. Then Amy asked if I was cross about her staying away the previous week – did I 'miss her'. I said that I thought she might be punishing me – 'it was like keeping her brother waiting' but I also said that I thought she might be the one who misses out. After I thought that this was too much like scolding.

She chose a black pen. Her brother came on Thursday but didn't go and see her 'instead he saw the bus and got on'. She repeated this and I commented on how very angry she sounded 'furious' – 'Yes' she said, 'what was your word – furious – wouldn't you be?' She began drawing a grid in black – 'looks like a mat or could be a window'. I then suggested 'a window to a prison'. Amy then described a film – 'This daughter who is put into a handicapped hospital, left there by her mother and was then murdered by this man – they don't know who – wandering about'. This was linked to a man who others say roams the hospital. I asked if the man had come for her brother – but this seemed all wrong. Amy accepted that the daughter was like her. Her brother, she told me, 'when he does come doesn't stay long – well he stays until 3.30 but he keeps thinking about the bus and his tea' She wanted to know if he will visit regularly when she moves to the hostel. I said that she had been fighting with her brother for a long time. She draws a roof with cross-hatching for 'tiles'. I suggested that we could think about why it might be difficult for her brother to visit her, why he got on the bus. But Amy focussed on her anger – 'wouldn't you be'. Then she turned to her younger brother who died in the hospital and the 'neglect' of her mother and father. She has two brothers that are alive – 'The other one being worse', he 'could have me at home but I will pee on chairs, the furniture and the bed – Martin doesn't say this when he takes me out to a café'. I then said that her feelings arose because she had been abandoned in the hospital and neglected and that I thought the murderous man was really herself – her feelings. She listened and said 'Yes' but this also frightened her. She said she had been here for 45 years.

I pointed to the drawing and said how there was a roof at the top and a carpet or a mat on the floor but 'nothing in between'. I then said that maybe she felt she had been treated like a doormat. She agreed 'yes I have – wouldn't you feel like that' (Figure 9).

I seemed to be keen to provide interpretations and words for Amy to use in this session. Did she want me to be disgusted with her account of sexual activity with Dennis? This reminds me of the swill bin of Session 51 and seems to be another form of transgression. Perhaps she is saying that this is preferable to attending Art Therapy and that is why my 'scolding' appears. 'Furious' she likes as a word and she responds to my introduction of the idea of 'prison' to remind me that the hospital was a prison of sorts but also a dangerous place. The murderous man could relate to the sexual assault described in Session 14. I seem to want to effect a reconciliation in relation to her brother. However, Amy did listen carefully when I offered her the interpretation that the dangerous man could be related to her feelings. The idea of being 'treated like a doormat' arose because I was remembering the story about the abuse of a member of staff by the sister who was 'wiping the floor with her' (Session 48).

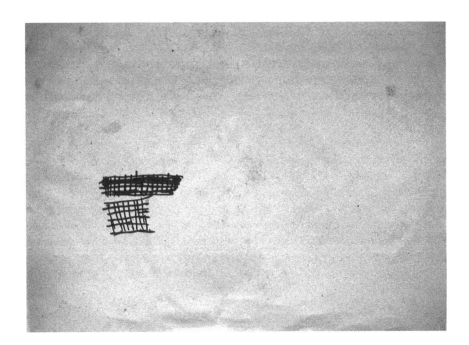

Figure 9 Roof and window or two grids. Felt tip on A2 paper.

The bottom grid is a 'mat or a window' and the top grid is the roof 'tiles'. But the two black grids on the grubby paper (see Session 39 where torn and grubby paper is used) when related to the material of the session, exemplify Amy's despair, her struggle with her brother, the pain of her abandonment, and the pain that arises from 45 years of institutional life.

Fifty-Eight Session

Amy came on time and stood near to me. 'Mrs Thatcher', she began, 'They've got to get rid of her now – will they get somebody better?' I suggested that maybe she was wondering if I was now 'getting rid' of her as she was going to the hostel, 'would I get somebody better?'. 'Yes' Amy responded 'I don't know will you?' Following this exchange she talked about her mother, 'I mustn't talk about her must I disturb the dead – she's dead now – I don't want to disturb her'. I said, 'it sounds like you're making amends'. She didn't understand 'amends' and I explained, and this lead her to talk about feeling guilty because she threw a hairbrush at her mother and 'poured water over her new blue coat' and her mother chased her with a knife and gave her 'snuff' which damaged her brain. Her parents blamed each other when her brother with 'golden hair' died. 'I didn't cry when my mother died – that's awful' Amy said. Her mother promised her a sister but she did not have one. I then said how she felt that her mother wanted to murder her and rob her of her children – brothers and sisters. She asked for an explanation and I went over my thinking, emphasising the death of her brother, and the sister who was promised but did not appear. Amy said 'Yes I see what you mean'. I then suggested that maybe her mother and her father had their own problems. Amy told me that they were 'fighting all the time – rowing terrible – I couldn't stand it'.

As she was speaking she was drawing a 'square'. Her father had taught her how to draw it 'he could be kind but was strict – going to bed without a hot water bottle when freezing on holiday'. The square was 'a square box'. I thought she had said swear box.

Mrs Thatcher has enabled Amy to think about her relationship not only with me but also her mother. She cannot talk too much about her mother because her mother lives as a disturbing image in her mental life. The story of the blue coat and her mother's retaliation provides some further explanation of the origins of the disturbance that haunts her, and Amy seems to appreciate my Kleinian interpretation in this session. Amy tells us, through the use of the drawing, that she did learn something from her kind, but strict father, who left her cold and freezing when on holiday. I misheard 'the square box' as 'the swear box', but then I did think of the box as containing difficult material, feelings or thoughts that have been buried or repressed.

Fifty-Ninth Session

She was late because she had got to the canteen late. Barry and Jim were 'jealous' and she complained that Barry was 'dopey' – 'he keeps on about the hostel – gets mixed up'. The night nurse told Barry to 'piss off – not nice is it?' Amy used a yellow crayon. I asked her if she was anxious in relation to the move to the hostel and I suggested that could be the reason for coming late, that she didn't want to think about it. 'No I didn't' she said and her drawing she described as 'a square – could be a window'.

Maybe the thought of spending her life with Barry was not what she would ideally choose. Being told to 'piss off' reminds me of the getting rid of Mrs Thatcher, this is what the hospital is doing getting rid of the bad Mother Amy, and Barry. Amy enjoys Barry's dependency, and Jim's jealousy, but she wants to defend Barry against hostile staff. Thinking about the hostel is difficult, especially if you might not want to go. The square, previously a box, now becomes a window, looking out at the world beyond the hospital.

Sixtieth Session

Amy tells me about a girl who is greedy, always wanting tea – then she laughs – and admits, without me saying anything – that it is her who is really greedy and always wanting tea. She draws a house using several different colours. Barry she tells me is worried all the time and gets the dates wrong. I notice that she appears agitated; she is taking the tops off the pens and then immediately replacing them. I say, 'well Barry is worried, but what about your feelings – you're saying nothing about your feelings, but you seem agitated'. She says that a woman in the shop had said 'a lot of people will miss you Amy' and I suggested that she will miss her friends. She told me that she was kept awake all night long 'in her sleep making noises – aggravating in her sleep'. In the drawing, she was 'searching for the white door'.

I wasn't sure who it was 'in her sleep' that was making noises, and where the 'aggravation' was coming from. Maybe I was intended to think of it simply as a disturbing dream that resulted in a very restless and difficult night. Other patients or residents do make noises and the noises could be linked to 'the deaf and dumb girl crying in her bed' (see Session 51). The white door we had seen previously (Figure 4, Session 10, p63) is a door that is very difficult to locate – it is the door out of the hospital and into the hostel. Its whiteness, like the white strokes or lines on white paper, is the noise of desperation 'aggravating' her sleep, perhaps.

Sixty-First Session

Amy asks, 'should I come or go to the party?' She tells me she is worried about aids as she has been 'rubbing Dennis's cock'. 'Can I get aids from him?' she asks. I asked her if she understood what Michele had said to her, and if Dennis had put his penis into her vagina. 'Yes Michele said that – do you mean if you go all the way?' After going to the woods with Dennis she had to clean mud off her shoes before going into the ward. I asked her if she felt dirty after seeing Dennis. She said 'Yes – another girl had told somebodies mother that Dennis was a rapist'. She had to clean her shoes and wasn't allowed out in the evening because she had been going to the woods. The staff 'took the mickey' out of her. She asked, 'Is it right that if you had a baby over 40 it would be a mongol – I read one about a woman of 72 who had a baby'.

Amy was drawing a house in red as she spoke, 'Dennis got two other girls pregnant – in the hostel there'll be another Dennis (a nurse)'. Amy admitted that she would miss Dennis and that it wasn't the same with Barry. I suggested to her that she found Dennis exciting, in the woods etc. – 'I do', she laughed, 'I'll miss you too and you'll miss me won't you'. I agreed with her statements. The house she was drawing 'could be the hostel' and it was important that it had a 'chimney and a letter box'. Before the end of the session, she added a second house.

If she is not going to get aids from Dennis, then her phantasy is that Dennis will provide her with a baby – if not now then in some imagined future. Is a baby possible now she is wondering. Then in a more sober mood, Amy recognizes that going to a hostel entails loss. The need for the chimney and the letter box in her drawing indicates the importance she attaches to her sexual life with Dennis, which was diminished and ridiculed by others.

Sixty-Second Session

She had spent a week in the sick ward and wanted to know why I did not visit her. She talked of people dying – a woman the same age as herself. She felt she could die from what she had. The nurse did not believe her when she talked about her oedema. Amy emphasised that she was going to go to the hostel in March and she asked if I would visit her. I said that I would pay her a visit. 'There was a resident who said he wasn't going to die – everybody dies no matter how strong you are', she told me. The painting she was producing she called 'strokes' and I related it to her mother. Amy responded by saying 'couldn't help it could she'.

I didn't visit Amy in the sick ward because I did not know that she was there. My assumption was that she had decided to miss a session. After this session, I did regret not making an inquiry. Amy now feels that the 'strokes' are coming her way.

Sixty-Third Session

She was late as she had been going to the farm with Dennis and the Nurses were rude to her about it. She said that she would be 'glad to get out of here – this hospital'. Dennis, she said, 'didn't treat people nicely – stripping them naked and leaving them in the cold – to get cold'. Amy asked if she should start the work or if was it too late. I linked Dennis's behaviour to my behaviour and suggested that she had felt let down by me left out in the cold (on the sick ward). 'That's just in your mind' she responded.

Dennis's stripping people and 'leaving them in the cold' does feel like another kind of abandonment. But what may have been important for Amy was to have some fun with Dennis, on the farm, before she has to leave, despite what the nurses say. Getting out of the hospital is still very much desired in this session, is it all too late?

Sixty-Fourth Session

I saw Amy in the sick ward. She was very pale in the hospital bed, with sunken cheeks. She was coughing, her speech was delivered in fragments, and it was difficult to be sure of what she was saying. Amy was clear that she wanted to go with the social worker as planned, with Barry, to a hostel. Amy was also worried that she would lose her place in the Art Therapy and that I would tell her off for not coming. I tried to reassure her that she would not lose her place. Then she began drift in and out of consciousness and I ended the visit, after an hour, by suggesting that she should make herself as comfortable as possible and try to get some sleep.

The nursing staff later the next day reported to me that, on the evening of my visit, Amy had 'drifted off into a coma' and that she died shortly after.

I attended Amy's funeral. Amy was very popular with the residents and the staff of the hospital, and the small hospital Chapel was full. Dennis, Barry and Jim with the stick were there. There was an air of celebration and during the service, the Chaplain reminded the congregation of Amy's history of winning art competitions. But Amy's brothers did not attend.

When I learnt that her brothers were not there I began to think about my Father who separated from my Mother and left the family home when I was 6 years old. My brother wrote to me when I was 21 to tell me that he had been killed in a road accident. I did not feel that I could attend his funeral because at the time I was stationed in Germany. This was to be my excuse at any rate. I learned later from other siblings that nobody from the family attended his funeral. This abandonment, by the family, at the moment when a life might be celebrated appeared to me, later in life, to be particularly bad.

I began to realise, sometime after, that my experiences with Amy were critical to my personal development and awareness. I regretted not being more active in Amy's life outside of the therapeutic space, for example in the resettlement process, but I found the staff meetings around resettlement depressing, especially as they often ended in wrangles about finance. I did think that my proper role was to provide a consistently available space and material for Amy to find expression and develop her thinking. This idea consoles me, in my loss.

Final Brief Comment

Meltzer and Harris Williams describe a psychoanalytical model of the mind, 'marked by the progression Freud-Abraham-Klein-Bion' which 'shattered the assumption of unity' and which, with Bion, placed 'its emphasis on the mind as an instrument for thinking about emotional experiences' (Meltzer and Harris Williams 1988, p7). It is, accordingly 'the creation of idiosyncratic symbols, as opposed to the manipulation of conventional signs' that 'marks the watershed between growth of the personality and adaptation' (Meltzer and Harris Williams 1988, p14).

In Art Therapy, the 'idiosyncratic symbol' is the product of the hand at work on material in a setting where the other is present. However we are required to give consideration to words, which are present when the hand is in use, and we want to think about how these words, of the client and the therapist, might relate to what is visual and haptic. This dialectic can be experienced as a never-ending research process (see Skaife 2000).

In her art production, Amy was sometimes confident and decisive, at other times hesitant and in doubt, leaving work unfinished. She always worked from a standing position, and her use of her hands in gesture, and in engagement with materials, was usually accompanied by speech. I want to now bring the reader's attention to two house images, her use of clay and plasticine, and the drawing of 'strokes' and 'lines' so that we can consider hand-use and speech together as both communication and mental activity, that is thinking.

Two Houses

Amy begins her Art Therapy with a house and figure, Session 1 (Figure 3, p57). The house and the figure together can be regarded as a self-presentation, which serves as a demonstration of her independence from her mother, and an exhibition of her ability. My comment on the initial absence of a door may have undermined her confidence and serves as a partial explanation for the anxiety that appears in her verbal imagery, which was at odds with the painting. What's important to note is that the house, and her verbal imagery, was a response to the new situation, the new venture, Art Therapy in the smaller of the two studio spaces, with the new art therapist; a man as opposed to a woman, previously.

An incomplete house was drawn in Session 57, further on and close to the end of our time together (see Figure 9, p91). Amy explained why she missed the previous session; she had been buying a 'low grade' 'tea in the canteen'. She then related how she agreed to push her finger into her boyfriend's bottom. She was particularly angry with her brother for coming to the hospital but not meeting with her, and she also spoke of the neglect of her mother and father. I was more interpretative than usual in this session, mostly I think because I was in touch with the strength of her anger, not because I had any helpful insight.

Amy was clearly seeking to find an expression for her desires, and for her anger, in a world which had become impoverished and soiled. Death threatens in the shape of the angry murderous man and after 45 years in the hospital it becomes increasingly difficult to hold on to hope. The coherent image of the house presented at the beginning, in Session 1, has been lost. We may regard this later, unfinished house, as the product of a regression, but it is the product of an increase in her capacities to recognise the feeling. The two black grids on the grubby paper are a translation of her despair into material form, and it emerges in an intersubjective space where there is a communication to and from another.

Clay

In Session 2 Amy used the clay. She worked while standing, as usual, producing gestures while she talked. She appeared reluctant to handle the clay. She made many arm and hand movements above the lump on the table, without making contact. When she had shaped the clay it was difficult for her to decide what was being made, a bird, dog and cat, or balls? She gave the bird some eyes but production ended in a 'sausages'. I was struck by her direct eye-level gaze which was particularly assertive and after I answered her question in relation to my parents Amy was able to give an account of her family and herself, a verbal self-presentation, which could be compared to the visual self-presentation, in the previous session, Session 1. Although I seemed to be impressed by this verbal self-presentation I remained aware of her ambivalence and uncertainty which was implied in her reference to 'long time over breakfast', but more directly, on a feeling level, through her response to the clay, especially the movements related to use and non-use. I was thinking that the work was going to be difficult and I was not yet fully committed to this work – in this sense the ambivalence Amy communicated was shared. Nevertheless something was, with the making, in a continuous process of transformation, even if it could not be definitively named until the end of the session, and what do 'sausages' indicate?

Lines and Strokes

'Lines' and 'strokes' as Amy called them, were often produced from Session 13 through to Session 53. They appeared in small groups, sometimes with other imagery, often with a 'box' or an attempt at a 'box'. 'Strokes' appear in the drawing of herself on a high chair as a small child, they also appear in the Jekyll and Hyde drawing. When making a 'stroke', or 'line', Amy often gestured with her crayon, pencil, pen or oil pastel above the paper, and in this way her pattern of speech, movement and hesitation in engaging with the material element replicated her use of clay.

In Session 12 Amy, pleased with herself for being angry with her brother, was decisive in her use of crayons. She drew shapes, circles, squares, a triangle, diamond and a star. She talked about suspected food and 'poison', and asked about 'purgatory'. If others thought that she deserved to be poisoned, Amy was sure, herself, that she was going to heaven. The 'lines' that appeared in the next Session 13 were altogether different. She used a white crayon on white paper, making several marks or lines. After deciding to use the white crayon on brown paper, she returned to using the same crayon on the white paper again. Finally, she chose a pink crayon to use on the white paper. She had been for an EEG and wanted to know what was wrong with her head. Amy knew that she was 'a bit slow' but she was taken advantage of. She mentioned a father who murdered his son and then ended the session by drawing a box which was imagined to contain tools and a handkerchief. Everything seems enigmatic in this session. The white line on the white paper, in its repetition, does seem to be signifying an invisibility. It is only partially like the white door that is difficult to see. The white door seems to be more about finding an entrance to a house. There was a reference to sickness in this session and Amy expressed a preference for dying in her sleep, and the presence of impairment, disease and death, could be characterised as that invisible element in life, given form by the white line.

Amy did, on occasion, make direct links between the 'lines' or 'strokes' to her words, for instance when Amy reports that Dennis strikes her with a piece of wood across her neck, she produces a 'stroke'. In Session 30 Amy links the 'strokes' in the Mr Hyde drawing to the death of her mother who died because of 'strokes'.

In Session 40 Amy is anxious that she may not be able to recover consciousness if she goes unconscious. She tries to watch the film 'The Ten Commandments' but a cleaner changes the channel. Her mother had urged her to watch this film and now a message is lost. Four 'mauve' lines in this session refer to a colour that is Amy's by choice, the colour that her Mother does not like (see Session 1).

I now think of the lines and strokes as marks that, *by themselves*, may not directly communicate as signifiers, they cannot generate an interpretant, or be translated in any secure way, but they relate to thought processes, and communications, dispersed across speech, movement and the engagement with materials.

Damarell (2011) researched the use of hands, and words, during image-making with people with learning disabilities, using video. He identifies the presence of 'proto-declarative' pointing with the marker, where the participant draws attention to the observer to 'important material in the maker's imagery'. He then describes 'positional movements above the marking surface' which Damarell translates; firstly as a 'gesture to be made in relation to the image maker herself'; and secondly as an 'indication of conscious contemplation and action'. Next Damarell describes 'shaping movements' and a combination of 'positioning' and 'shaping'. Shaping movements he observed were often 'graceful and sensual in their execution' and Damarell hypothesised that positioning is predominantly conscious, whereas shaping has 'its origins in unconscious functions' (Damarell 2011, p134). The talk was often directed towards sharing knowledge during the marking, Damarell observes, and was linked to the imagery in this way. Self-talk could be about the material element, the colours used, but also the construction of pictures, and Damarell linked self-talk to the movements he identified. Damarell ends by stressing the importance of physicality in 'relation to the creative process' 'even before a mark has been made' (Damarell 2011, p138). This research provides us with a very good description of movements we can witness when an individual is making use of art materials, and sharing the products of this activity with others, and we can see that movement is closely related to the sharing of visual interest, speech, and material engagements.

Damarell's researches are supported by cognitive researches on gesture in relation to speech. For instance, McNeill (2005) argued that gesture could be understood as a 'material carrier' .... '*the actual motion of the gesture itself*, is a dimension of thinking' (p98, emphasis in original). Clark (2013) argues that the 'physical act of gesturing' is '*part of a unified thought-language hand system*' and gesture is a 'material structure that is available to both speaker and listener' (Clark 2013, p258 & p259, emphasis in the original). This would suggest that separating physical movement, and the production of the visual, from the verbal, in an analysis, could be counterproductive, since all three *together* represent an attempt to process thought and feeling to find expression.

Briefly I now want to consider two Psychoanalysts who have wanted to establish the beginnings of thought and feeling which finds expression. Firstly Kristeva (1982) who proposes that mental life originates with the body, and its relation to the caregiver. Kristeva suggests that in phantasy at an unconscious level, the infant may murder her mother, in a cannibalistic manner through oral aggression. This murderous impulse is presented as a refusal of matriarchal power, upon which the infant is dependent, and serves as an attempt to separate. This results in the emergence of the 'abject'. 'The abject is not an object facing me which I name or imagine' it is a 'jettisoned object... radically excluded'. There is a 'weight of meaninglessness' attached to the abject 'which crushes me' but the 'abject and abjection are my safeguards' (Kristeva 1982, p1 & p2). Kristeva describes the 'abject' as 'the violence of mourning for an 'object' that has always already been lost' (Kristeva 1982, p15).

We saw that Amy was haunted by a sometimes murderous mother, who she repudiates. After forgetting about Amy in the shop her mother is denied. The murderous Mr Hyde, who the good Dr Jekyll, cannot rid himself of, troubles Amy, and Kristeva does associate the abject with an aspect of the super-ego which radically unsettles the stability of the subject. The 'strokes', and 'lines', in their visibility, and invisibility, and their link to her mother's death, can be imagined as the troubling absence at the core of the 'abject', which we could argue appears in different guises throughout the therapy, for instance as the 'wicked witch' and the 'murderous man', although the latter could also refer to a traumatic experience – the rape in Session 14.

Kristeva's reconstruction of a beginning in which the infant responds to the caregiver who provides, but also overwhelms, can be compared with Laplanche's (1999) view. Laplanche proposes to *begin* with the other, the parental figures; it is the other who is constitutive in relation to the infant's psychic life, especially in the form of an unconscious, which the subject experiences as alien. The 'unconscious is only maintained in its radical alterity by the other person... in brief, by seduction' (Laplanche 1999, p71). Laplanche does not intend us to think of the unconscious as the other 'simply implanted in me' but it is in the form of a message addressed to the infant 'to someone with no shared interpretative system' (p79). The message contains the enigma of the other's unconscious. The message is described as both social and sexual, and in development, the individual attempts to both 'master', and 'translate, these ... traumatizing messages' (p165). Laplanche presents this as a continuous task throughout life, and old translations get re-translated. Memories, and fragmentary memories, are 'shot through with enigmatic parental messages' he suggests (p161). In relation to mourning, Laplanche argues, that the parental message 'has never been adequately understood, never listened to enough' (p254). Mourning is rarely without 'regret or remorse for not having been able to speak with the other enough, for not having heard what he had to say' (Laplanche 1999, p254).

This last idea of Laplanche's certainly resonates with my own experience of mourning, and I find myself now thinking about the loss of a letter from my father in adolescence. But what about Amy? There is of course the ten commandments which contains a message from her mother, and after the 'stroke' her mother could not speak. Amy does mention lost letters, and not having the time to write letters, but throughout the Art Therapy there was a continuous attempt by Amy to reconnect with both her parental figures but especially her mother, and we can think of her as remembering and attempting different translations of the enigmatic parental message – a 'working-through under the power of the originary enigmatic situation' (Laplanche 1999, p98).

The Larger Other

There is a larger Other present in the therapeutic setting, namely the institution in its discursive practices. Amy understands the Art Therapy as work, since art making in other workshops, regarded by the staff as recreational, is presented to her as work. She says she should be retired. Amy is obliged to follow the routines of Art Therapy, just as she has to follow the routines of the nursing staff; she has to accept that staff have holidays. Staff behave illegally; they don't stick to their agreements. She is subject to abuse from the staff when she is 'slow', and that is present when she is often in opposition to the institutional power to which she is subject. She wants to know what does the institution really think, what does it mean to be 'mental', what is exactly wrong with her head? She cannot get a satisfactory answer to this question, and she cannot effect any change in her situation but must rely on staff – and be patient and face disappointment in relation to a move from the hospital. Amy is not well and is aware of the proximity of death, she sees others dying, and how can she wait, she has already wasted 45 years. Although her brother visits he serves as a reminder of her abandonment. Amy is aware of my limits, like the dentist I cannot 'take the pains away', and, when I insist on the boundaries of my practice, I can be seen as cruel, not unlike 'Bullet'.

Amy was obliged to digest the experience of abandonment and incarceration which brings with it a particular form of alienation. When I remember my time with Amy and consider this his/herstory I have produced, I think of Amy as mourning her multiple losses, or attempting and failing to mourn, becoming melancholic, but then attempting recovery, whilst despairing.

Kierkegaard's Anticlimacus describes for us many forms of despair. He tells us that despair is ubiquitous, there is, perhaps no one, who

> is not to some extent in despair, in whose inmost parts there does not dwell ...
> a discord, an anxious dread of an unknown something, or of a something he
> does not even dare to make acquaintance with, a dread of a possibility of life,
> or dread of himself.
>
> Kierkegaard (1941, p32)

Amy's despair could be understood as the despair of possibility. 'When a human existence is brought to the pass that it lacks possibility, it is in despair'. If there is only that necessity which is imposed upon me, then hope may not be possible. For 'the self to become freely itself'... 'possibility and necessity are equally essential'.

Possibility can take the form of 'wishful, yearning' or 'melancholy fantastic'; the difficulty is in finding hope that can be related to existing necessity (Kierkegaard 1941, p53 & p57).

Dr Jekyll and Mr Hyde ends with Jekyll's 'Full Statement of the Case' where he describes himself as suppressing his 'gayety of disposition' to achieve respectability, a desire to carry his 'head high, and wear a more than commonly grave countenance before the public' (Stevenson 1964, p97). Thus he begins to despair in his dissociation between a desire for some form of transgressive liberty that is curtailed by a high seriousness, and an absolute duty to others. There was a requirement for Amy to assume the appearance of a compliant self, an adaptable individual who would not be difficult to rehabilitate into the community, one who could be presentable as respectable and ordinary. Her transgressive desires were to be left behind with Dennis in the hospital. This generates a despair of not being one-self. This despair, which is protest and sustains, is affectively present in the production of white lines on white paper.

References

Clark, A. 2013. Gesture as Thought? Chapter IV. In: Radman, Z. (Ed.) *The Hand, an Organ of the Mind.* Massachusetts Institute of Technology, Massachusetts, pp. 255–268.

Damarell, B. 2011. Shaping Thoughts: An Investigation into the Cognitive Significance of Image-Making for People with Learning Disabilities. Chapter 5. In: Gilroy, A. (Ed.) *Art Therapy Research in Practice.* Peter Lang AG, International Academic Publishers, Bern, pp. 117–138.

Kierkegaard, S. 1941. *The Sickness unto Death.* Lowrie, W. (Trans.). Princeton University Press, Princeton, NJ.

Kristeva, J. 1982. *Powers of Horror – An Essay on Abjection.* Roudiez, L. S. (Trans.). Columbia University Press, New York.

Laplanche, J. 1999. *Essays on Otherness.* Fletcher, J. (Ed.). Routledge, London and New York.

McNeill, D. 2005. *Hand and Mind.* University of Chicago Press, Chicago.

Meltzer, D. & Harris Williams, M. 1988. *The Apprehension of Beauty – The Role of Aesthetic Conflict in Development, Violence and Art.* The Clunie Press for the Roland Harris Educational Trust, Strath Tay.

Skaife, S. 2000. Keeping the Balance: Further Thoughts on the Dialectics of Art Therapy. In: Gilroy, A. & McNeilly, G. (Eds.) *The Changing Shape of Art Therapy – New Developments in Theory and Practice.* Jessica Kingsley Publishers, London and Philadelphia.

Stevenson, R.L. 1964. *Dr.Jekyll and Mr. Hyde.* Airmont Publishing Co., Inc. New York.

Chapter 5

Edward

PART 1

Introduction

Edward (a pseudonym), a 50-year-old man who was a resident of Hospital B, attended weekly individual sessions of Art Therapy with me for six years. We met in the larger Art Therapy Room which was used for group work. There were three large tables in the centre of the space, with six chairs, a plan chest and shelves, and cupboards under the sink – see Chapter 3, Figure 2. The bay window gave Edward and me a view over a green Meadow with trees in the distance. It was a well-designed light studio space, formal and instrumental in feel, rather than homely. I did add some large curtains over the observation window which softened the space. Edward would have known the building, previously from the outside, as a mortuary.

When providing Art Therapy for Edward it was Klein's thinking that influenced my working practices, which were then very much in the process of development. I was supported in clinical supervision by a therapist whose practice was informed by object relations theory, and to help me in self-understanding I also began to attend, three times weekly psychoanalytical psychotherapy delivered by a Kleinian therapist.

Kleinian theory stresses that understanding of the other is coloured by phantasy and feeling, and the development of internal objects, but the nature of the other is critical in this. Relations at the beginning of life to the other, and of necessity to the outer world which frames the dyad, are for Klein determined by an early dependency which is presented as characteristic of the human condition. I found that appreciating the conflictual element in dependency to be important in appreciating the relationship that Edward and myself were often struggling to establish, between ourselves. Dependency here refers not only to the client's or resident's dependencies but also the dependencies of the art therapist. In addition, I grew aware, while providing Art Therapy in Hospital B, of the centrality of phantasy, phantasy as an unconscious element in our mental activity and in our social lives.

The case study ends with a discussion and a summary in which I explore other theoretical frames. This element of the case presentation is closer to my current

DOI: 10.4324/9781003360056-6

thinking and represents a reflection at a distance. I have attempted to give an honest account of my practice in this study, and for me, the value of revisiting this case is that enables me to be self-critical and think about the mistakes I made.

Methodology

I regard the research element in this study as essentially heuristic, that is I am seeking to discover. In particular, through rewriting the case, revisiting the imagery, and producing a reflection I am trying to gain a clearer picture of the relationship that developed in the Art Therapy, and the intersubjective achievements that emerged in the setting, immersed as it was in the practices of Hospital B. What value did Art Therapy have for Edward and what was he able to gain from the sessions? That might be the question.

In presenting the case afresh, I will first make use of institutional documents to give an account of the referral. The hospital documents give us some limited understanding of how Edward was produced as a subject with intellectual disabilities and mental health difficulties. Focussed as they often were on the management of aggressive behaviours and the antipathy and difficulties that Edward had in using speech to explore feeling, the documents reflect staff understanding and frustration, but they were also suggestive in relation to the problems that the therapist might anticipate. As well as suggesting future problems the documents include an institutional demand, addressed to the art therapist, that Edward should be understood as in need of help to express his feelings in a form that enables others to appreciate his motivations and understanding. From an institutional perspective, a verbal communication of some sort would be preferred, but in relation to visual expression, it is hoped that the art therapist might serve as some kind of translator, and that Edward would thereby be enabled to give an account of himself.

After this brief exploration of the hospital documents, I will present Edward's art production and my reflections that arose from viewing the art work, mostly drawings, that Edward left behind in the department. Edward produced approximately 30–35 images in each hourly session. He attended weekly and he left behind, in the department almost 5,000 drawings. The drawings were made with oil pastels, or crayons, and were often made from lines of different colours. I photographed some of his work and some photographs have been reproduced in this study for readers, so that an appreciation of his use of colour can be seen. Other photographs were used as a basis for making traces so that I could present them as black and white drawings. This tracing was motivated by cost but also to gain clarity in relation to the line, as some of the photographs had been taken in poor light.

Looking at the drawings entailed a graduated repetitive exposure, that is to say that it was a looking as the work was produced and emerged in the sessions, but also immediately after the session in the department, when writing notes. During the note writing, I would record Edward's comments, if any, about the work, and also my own verbal responses to the imagery in the sessions. Later I periodically undertook retrospective reviews of the work, often while photographing the work.

Exposure to the imagery in this way was visually stimulating and I was then able to recapture something of the emotional element present during my time with Edward.

There is no numerical analysis of imagery in my research, instead, my relation to Edward and his art production, encouraged me to search for repetitions amongst the drawings, repetitions and variations that could be regarded as an indication of a development. As I identified themes I noticed that they could be enlarged into narratives, and this in turn affected my subsequent search and further discovery.

I have produced some reflection on production processes and the particularities of some individual images are then explored in more detail. My comment in relation to imagery might be regarded as ekphrastic, in that I attempt to provide a written account of a visual experience. This writing is ostensive in nature. It is supported by an illustration to enable the reader to follow my thought processes, but also, like all such ekphrastic writing, it is intended to be descriptive but is unavoidably interpretative. Comments that Edward made in relation to his drawings are included.

Following the exploration of art production, in Part 3 I will present a narrative of the sessions constructed from process notes that I made of the sessions as the therapy progressed. I have used notes that have some relation to the visual material discussed in the analysis of the drawings, and I have used notes that include reference to material and verbal exchanges that the analysis of the drawings does not engage with. There are gaps in this narrative. We met weekly, and the therapeutic process, as it is presented, does not represent in any way a total account of the case – if such a thing were possible. I have numbered each session that appears in my narrative consecutively but added month and year so that the reader can appreciate where the gaps fall. I have tried to give a clear picture of the therapist, myself, at work and include interventions which I now find questionable and, to some degree, embarrassing. Comment and reflection which I have inserted into this section is influenced by the frame, or the theoretical constructs, that motivated my interventions and shaped my note writing. Later reflections that emerged during the rewrite of the study which was originally submitted for an M.A. appear in italics. My hope is that this section of the study will give the reader an account of how verbal exchanges, which were mostly initiated by myself (the therapist), were related to the production of drawings, events, and movement in the therapeutic relationship.

My verbal interventions often took the form of questions or comments related to the production of drawings, and were sometimes interpretative. I wanted to encourage language, but as will be seen Edward's use of language was limited, especially in the early sessions, sometimes he echoed my comments, and, apart from 'Yes Mister' and 'No Mister', he usually actively resisted encouragement, or pressure in respect of speech. In contrast, Edward did, as he grew in confidence, label his drawings and occasionally he spontaneously introduced imaginative narrative content in the form of verbal reference to actions, not necessarily visually present in the image we looked at together. This narrative content was brief and associations were limited, but it did indicate that language had some importance in Edward's art production and thinking.

Hospital Documents

Edward, at 50 years of age, was referred to the Art Therapy Department by a concerned Consultant Psychiatrist. Edward often disappeared from view during the day, successfully avoiding the surveillance of the hospital staff, but after being found on the central reservation of a busy nearby motorway it was felt that something should be done, especially as he showed no 'apparent appreciation of the danger' that he confronted. It had not been possible to learn from Edward how or why he placed himself in this dangerous situation. One theory was that it represented his response to the limits placed upon cigarettes, but since the staff could not engage Edward in talking about himself and his motivations, it was asked if it might be possible for Edward to explore his thinking and feelings in Art Therapy, especially as he had shown some liking for drawing.

The hospital file contained little information about Edward. It was recorded that he had some minor fits at the age of 6 and developed some 'peculiar grimacing' later in his childhood. The suggestion here is that there were some organic and neurological events shaping his development. The files also produce Edward as a psychiatric casualty. At the age of 13, he was admitted to a large psychiatric hospital and three years later moved to the nearby 'mental handicap hospital'. Here, on admission, the diagnosis was recorded as Schizophrenia. At the time of referral to Art Therapy, 34 years after his admission to the hospital, Edward was prescribed Carbamazepine which is essentially an anticonvulsant used in the control of epilepsy. Although there was little contemporary evidence of epilepsy Carbamazepine was sometimes used in the hospital as adjunct to the management of 'challenging behaviour'. Edward was also prescribed Zuclopenthixol on a daily basis, which is an anti-psychotic medication.

In hospital B he was eventually assessed for a learning disability, and at the age of 34, on the Wechsler Intelligence Scale for Children (WISC) was given an overall IQ of 46. In the Peabody Picture Vocabulary Test he achieved a raw score of 56, and in his response to the Sequin Form Board test his 'mental age' was recorded as seven years. It is interesting that he was not assessed using the adult version of the WISC – which would suggest that he was already seen as child-like. Speech and Language therapists report that Edward was able to demonstrate a 'good level of functional understanding', that he can 'express himself well using language' and the complexity of Edward's 'expressive language is appropriate for his conversational need'. However, it is noted that Edward's ability to 'self-monitor his own language' has 'limitations' and he does not 'always appear to be fully aware of his own errors'. In conversation he is often reluctant to contribute and 'tends to follow his own train of thought' and it was thought that he did struggle to create 'appropriate novel sentences'.

Edward was an only child and the hospital files record Edward as being 'abusive' to parents, without reason he was unpredictably aggressive, attacking parents and smashing windows, breaking the TV and overturning furniture. The files describe him as having a 'double personality' and as being a 'moody shut-in' individual who 'frequently strikes and assaults other patients'. Nursing staff report that Edward is unable to tolerate the staff regulating his supply of cigarettes. He has, on several occasions, thrown furniture and threatened staff in a day care centre when demanding cigarettes. He is also reported to have thrown stones at cars belonging to hospital staff. Despite this record of antisocial violence, he did develop a good relationship with another patient, a Mr M. The staff thought that this was a sexual relationship. This relationship ended ten years before I met him. In day care settings it was thought that Edward was responding to auditory hallucinations, as he was seen talking to himself and placing his hands over his ears while silently screaming.

The files indicated that Edward's father visited regularly on Tuesdays and his mother every three weeks. However, at the time of his referral to Art Therapy his mother had ceased to visit and his father was visiting much more infrequently. His father suggested that Edward should be locked in, 'especially after dark'. Edward, the nursing staff reported, was often tense, when his father visited, and sometimes he wandered off while his father was on the ward, leaving his father to catch the bus back home. The parents moved their place of residence and did not want Edward to know where they now lived as they were afraid of his return. Edward's parents both died while Edward was attending Art Therapy, during the fifth year. This is recorded in 'resettlement meeting' minutes, but no clear date is given. Edward was friendly towards childhood neighbours who continued to visit him on occasions.

PART 2

Edward's Art Production

The referral, outlined above, resulted in Edward's engagement in Art Therapy. Edward's art work, or perhaps we should call it play as there was an imaginative engagement and an element of reverie in Edward's productive activity, consisted predominantly of drawing. The drawings are presented here through an assessment of what could loosely be regarded as content. The drawings were evidently pictures, and it was possible to decide what they were 'of' according to Edward's naming and sparse comments. As well as referential content, I will give some attention to the constructive drawing processes that enabled Edward to generate the immense amount of visual material that he slowly developed into narratives. These narratives enabled Edward to communicate verbally and in a more developed symbolic form. Lacan reflecting on the relation between the imaginary and the symbolic commented '…sometimes, for lack of images, some symbols don't see the light of day' (Lacan 1988, p88). Edward himself said 'another one of my drawings, sometimes they come out hard'.

When drawing Edward preferred using oil pastel on A2 sugar paper or cartridge. He worked rapidly and images carried the energy of his arm movements which, especially when he varied his colour, often produced a dramatic and expressive effect. By expressive here, I intend to convey the idea that the drawings were capable of transmitting feeling.

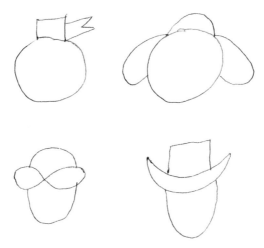

Figure 10 Drawings by the author of Edward's schema in relation to hats and faces.

The bulk of Edward's drawings were of faces and figures. A face, or head, when occupying the central area of the paper, was usually presented alone surmounted by a hat (See Figure 10).

The face could be represented by beginning the drawing with a circle to which a hat might be added, or a hat could be drawn first with the face added beneath using a semi-circular line, for example:

The 'donkey man' and the 'Judge' – top line left to right – two 'cowboys' on the bottom line, all identified by their hats.

Edward also developed a routine for the drawing of facial features (Figure 11). Here he made use of some simple graphic elements, or 'primitives' as described by Van Sommers (1984, p186), open circles, lines, cross-hatching, triangles, rectangles and ovals. Elements were combined and varied in simple constructions which allowed for a number of faces to be realised without the necessity of practicing and mastering fresh or complicated forms with each new pictorial problem.

Eyes might be represented by semi-circular marks with scribbled patches, or ovals containing circular scribble, or circles on occasions – see top line Figure 11. The nose was usually represented by a triangle but this could be varied with the addition of circular nostrils – see second line Figure 11. Mouths were also varied, giving the faces different kinds of expression – third line Figure 11. Ears were not always added to the faces but when present they were signified by the use of a simple bracket shape attached to the circle which denotes the contours of the face – bottom line.

Edward, we could say, had developed his own personal *visual* semiotic (see Atkinson 2002). Hats had a particular metonymic function, identifying a character, and Edward would point out the presence of these hats, which he once referred to as 'fighting hats'. The hat would stimulate him to describe action, for instance, in response to the hat identified as belonging to the 'French/donkey man', Edward

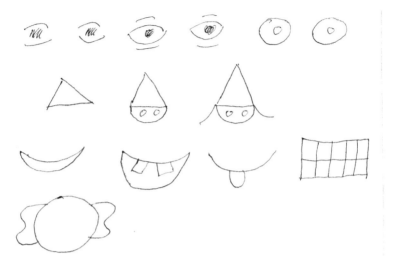

Figure 11 Drawing by the author of Edward's schema in relation to facial features, eyes, noses, mouths and ears.

says, 'dips his hat in the water to cool his head'. This action would not be visible since we only see the head of the 'French/donkey man' and his hat on his head in the drawing. Here we can see that the visual semiosis in the drawing, the production of iconic signs, generates verbal imagery and the beginnings of a narrative. When drawing Edward often moved quickly and confidently and a pile of drawings would rapidly appear on the table between the two of us. Although Edward was generally reluctant to speak the drawings did instigate speech, both on his part, and on the part of the therapist, and thereby more communication emerged.

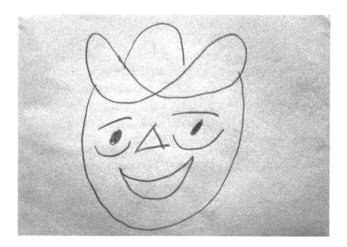

Figure 12 Oil pastel on A2 paper 'Cowboy'.

Edward often filled the paper with faces like this. They varied little in features or expression, and he was capable of producing 30 or more images of this kind in an hourly session.

Despite the repetition involved in the production of the cowboys, as shown in Figure 12, many of the rapidly sketched faces that Edward produced were full of live feeling, especially when using oil pastel and filling the central area of a sheet of A2 size using confident sweeps of his drawing arm (see Figures 13 and 14).

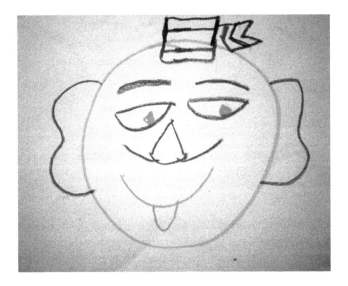

Figure 13 Oil pastel on A2. The 'Donkey man' or 'Frenchman'.

In Figure 13, the placement of the orange pupils of the eyes, and the raised eyebrows, gives the face a particular expression which is amplified in the context of the sticking out tongue – surprise, humour and delight perhaps. The face is certainly attentive, not just in terms of looking but also, the large ears suggest, listening. The hat, looking as it does like a railway signal, prompts *us*, the viewers, to take note. The lines attached to the nose could be a moustache, perhaps a French moustache. The colour contrasts animate the composition supplying life and energy to the whole.

In the pirate drawing (Figure 14) it is the terrible red eyes, the lines underneath that suggest tiredness, and the lines across the cheek area which may indicate scars or sunken cheeks, which carries the feeling. The pirate, his face under the skull and cross bones on his hat, looks directly out of the picture, challenging the viewer with his disturbing stare. I do feel that there is a vulnerability to this face. It is a Pirate who has suffered much. The difference between the two eyes suggests that he sees with one eye only.

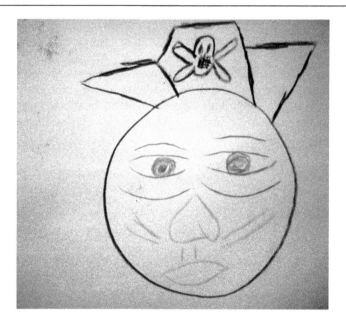

Figure 14 Pirate – Oil pastel on A2. A 'pirate'.

Faces with hats, which were always important to Edward, were sometimes given a rudimentary body, and when he chose to draw more slowly, and with more concentration, figures could become more elaborated, more complete with arms and hands, especially when the figure was involved in some action. Occasionally In some drawings stick men were used, for example when he wanted to populate a castle with soldiers. As I have already indicated cowboys were very popular with him and cowboy faces were sometimes repeated over and over again, without generating verbal associations. He did sometimes give an identity to the cowboy, for example 'Kit Carson' or 'Roy Rogers', but usually they remained anonymous. Cowboys were capable of action and could be shown carrying guns, or on a horse, or a stage coach, or near to Indians in their tents. The hats of the cowboys were varied a little. The headdresses of the Indians were differentiated by the number of feathers. As well as the round full face Edward drew, more rarely, a few profiles, for instance, 'a cowboy with a bandage on his nose'.

Many of the faces, and figures, in Edward's drawings could be described as cultural characters, which he named, for example; Charlie Chaplin, the Seven Dwarfs, Superman, Humpty Dumpty, Bob Hope, Educating Archie, Coco the Clown, Dick Barton, the Judge, and the Frenchman or Donkey Man. When Edward drew the Seven Dwarfs he usually concentrated on 'dopey'. He was sometimes reluctant to name 'dopey' instead he would then refer to 'the one before the end one'. Coco the clown and Charlie Chaplin as comedic outsiders may have shared some of the attributes of the dwarfs. 'Educating Archie' originates from a 1950s radio programme, as does 'Dick Barton'. Archie is a dummy who is educated by the ventriloquist who, notably, speaks through, or for him. Dick Barton, a detective, is often accompanied by 'Jock' who is a proletariat assistant who has connections with the underworld. The Frenchman or Donkey Man was linked by his hat to the teacher. The teacher appeared less frequently than the Frenchman and later, as my relationship with Edward progressed, the Donkey/French man became a figure riding donkeys or camels through the desert – I then began to think that Edward had seen a film about the French Foreign Legion. The Judge, Edward told me, 'knocks on the table with a hammer', he often appeared with the 'prisoner'. I did wonder if Edward was remembering a court appearance but he was unable to confirm this. He did confirm that that I was like the Judge when I knocked on the table to make him listen, insisting, as I sometimes did, that the drawing stops so that we could have a space in which we could look at the work together. There are of course other possible ways in which I might share attributes with the Judge, for instance in Judging Edward's work, and in starting and ending the sessions, sessions which might have had the semblance of a trial when I adopted an inter- rogative role. These cultural characters which Edward remained attached to reflect a working-class cultural consumption of radio and film available in the 1950s and early 1960s.

On rare occasions, Edward did draw figures more directly related to his experi- ences of others, father and mother for instance, and at one time he appeared to be attempting to portray friends or acquaintances in the hospital. Edward's drawings of his father were similar to his cowboys or Dick Barton, a smiling face with a simple hat. His mother was shown with a smiling face, without a hat, but with lots of scribbled hair around the circumference of the circular head.

The Castle

Edward drew a castle in the first session. This castle included sentries on the battle- ments, and three other figures, two of which were inside the castle. There was also 'a man playing a drum'. Five months after the start of Art Therapy, after he had begun to attend regularly, the castle appeared again. This second castle was drawn with the drawbridge up. Soldiers were placed on the battlements and the castle is shown being bombed by an aeroplane and shelled by a tank. Both the tank and the aeroplane are manned by soldiers and there is also a train arriving carrying soldiers (Figure 15).

The space provided by the paper, in this drawing, offers Edward the opportunity to stage a siege. There is a flag on the castle which suggests a Union Jack is be- ing flown, the same pattern is seen on the tail of the aeroplane, but here coloured in green. The aeroplane has both swastikas and roundels on its wings and body. On the battlements, some soldiers are drawn in red and some in green. Are some soldiers on the battlement attacking intruders? There are red soldiers on the aero- plane, which is dropping bombs, and red soldiers on the tank which is firing shells. A soldier in blue is descending by parachute. A pale blue train arrives at the wall

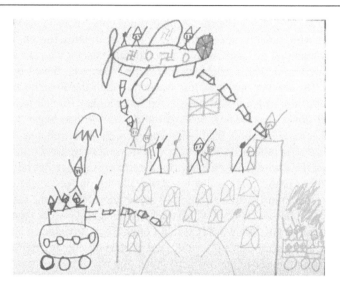

Figure 15 Felt Tip pen on A2. The castle (1).

filled with pale blue soldiers, or soldiers are escaping from the castle, as the train seems to moving towards the edge of the paper. The siege is full of action and it is difficult to know who defends the castle, what we can see is that there is a battle going on.

In year 3 Edward, after producing several pictures on the theme of guns, drew two men with guns on the battlements of the castle. There was no drawbridge or door to this picture. A man in a house in this session was putting a gun away in a drawer. Two months later the castle is again manned with soldiers, but without guns; however, the drawbridge is up. In the next castle picture, the castle has the square windows of a house, although it retains the drawbridge which is up. In the same month, the castle is drawn again, this time the drawbridge is replaced by a door with a handle, the number of flags increases and the soldiers disappear. At the end of this month the castle and a church become merged. There are two doors and a red drawbridge to this building, plus a tower with a cross on top. Armed soldiers on the castle do return the following month but a door has replaced the drawbridge.

Towards the end of the third year, Edward drew three figures on the battlements. Arms are outstretched, their hats are the hats of the 'donkey man', or 'French man'. This castle has three doors.

In the fourth year a dramatic action sequence is presented. (see Figure 16). A man makes his way through the door of the castle with the gun and then towards the battlements. It is the same figure that falls from the battlements with the gun in hand. Edward said 'been shot falling through the air'. There were two other drawings in this session that explored this theme, a drawing of a man with a gun, and another sheet which shows a man advancing towards a gate with a gun held out in front of him. Edward then said, 'going through the house to shoot someone'.

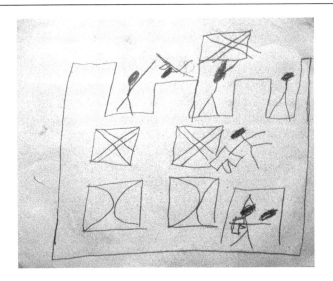

Figure 16 Pencil A2 – Castle (2).

After the Christmas holidays in the fifth year of therapy, the castle is drawn with three soldiers on the battlement with the drawbridge up. A soldier with a hat, Edward indicated, tells the others to stop firing. Three months later Edward draws a castle which has a fire blazing in a ground-floor room and a man appears descending a ladder, from a tower, while another figure is positioned just above the door. 'Man going up to the top of the castle – coming down to get a sword to attack man – he's in a hurry to get to the door' – Edward said.

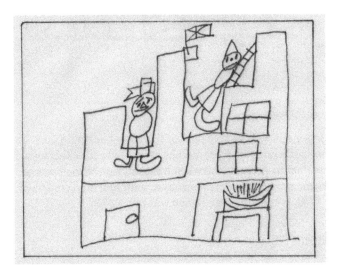

Figure 17 Original – Oil Pastel on pink A2 Paper – Castle (3) – tracing made by the author.

The figure above the door has the hat of the Donkey man/French man. There is still a danger from without as the man coming down the ladder is 'in a hurry' to attack a possible intruder – as Edward explained. The fire is an interesting addition to the castle theme and, on pink paper, suggests a warm interior, but see his comments below about the man who 'stokes up a big fire' in the castle.

The next castle that Edward produces is drawn with many more windows, the whole building broadened and extra towers added. In the Autumn a composite picture shows a castle, a house, a church, and a walking figure. The figure is a 'postman delivering a letter'. When I pointed to the different kinds of building Edward said that people prayed in the church and that he would prefer to live in a house. In the castle, he said, 'a man stokes up a big fire'.

At the end of the fifth year the castle is inhabited by children who are 'playing in the castle' – see Figure 18.

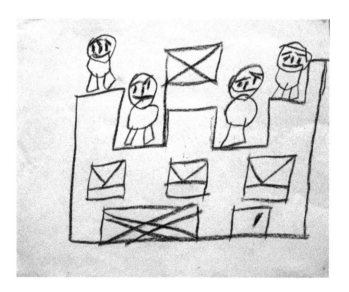

Figure 18 Black oil pastel on A2. The castle (4).

This castle appears to have both drawbridge (or a gate) and a door. The defensive aspects of the castle returned three months before the end of therapy when Edward was remembering his parents, and when a violent Iron Man appeared in his drawings he drew the old heavily defended castle with four soldiers armed. This castle had Gothic windows and the drawbridge was up.

The Windmill

The windmill makes its first appearance in the fifth month of therapy. Edward said that he saw a film about a windmill where 'a man gets inside – it starts working and goes round and round and he gets caught up'. This first windmill is coloured and simplified into rectangular sails and a triangular base. A month later it is drawn in green with a face in the centre looking alarmed. This strange face covers, or is covered by, what could be the base of the windmill in pink pastel – see Figure 19.

This appears to be a picture of the man 'caught up' in the windmill. Where the man's nose would be there seems almost to be another figure, possibly female, but it is difficult to know what Edward intended here. The large pink mound tempts me into a Kleinian interpretation and the semi-circular marks around the edge of the windmill and face suggest movement. The face does convey anxiety.

The windmill also appears in this same month with two men, positioned on either side of the windmill. The next time it is drawn it takes on the appearance of a house with sails and Edward says, 'it's a place where they sell pop – they don't sell tea'. The windmill next appears beside another tower with blue antennae which Edward names as a 'warning light'.

Just under a year after the first windmill, the windmill is shown as a place that requires protection. A cowboy is drawn standing beside the windmill and he is there, as Edward explains, to keep the robbers out, who robbed gold from the dungeon under the windmill. The windmill is drawn again four months later this time protected by a thick brown semi-circular wall and two guards. Three months later a man is standing next to the windmill, he has an unusual flower-like 'belly-button'.

At the beginning of the third year, a man is seen walking into the windmill while the same picture shows a boy with his hands raised, he wants some 'pop'. This picture also contains a house and an aeroplane. Later in the Spring of the third

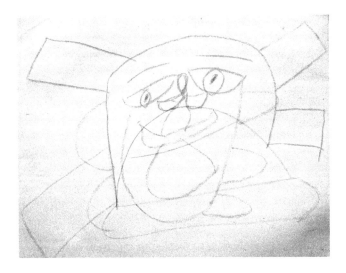

Figure 19 Oil pastel on A2. Windmill (1).

year Edward draws a house near to the windmill joined by a path which is accessed through a prominent double gate, or it is the same gate from both sides – see Figure 20.

The boy, bottom right, is 'running from the windmill' Edward said.

In a fresh picture in year 3, the house the windmill and the path which joins appear again. Underneath the mill and the house are 'a man and a boy'. 'The boy lived in the house and the man lived in the windmill', Edward told me.

The windmill appears alone in the next drawing of it, a month later, and Edward asks, 'the windmill is it still there? – by the forest? – you can get pop there 7p a bottle'. These associations continue in the Autumn when the windmill is roughly drawn, this time with a man standing beside it. 'He is the windmill man he drinks lemonade in the windmill through a blue and red straw' Edward says.

One month before the end of therapy the windmill is drawn with a cowboy outside and he recollected going on a trip with his parents to the windmill, 'when I was twelve', and getting 'pop inside'. The next windmill shows the 'Frenchman' inside the mill waving – see Figure 21.

Unlike the man 'caught up' (Figure 19) the Frenchman looks happy to be inside the windmill, waving and smiling, perhaps he is saying goodbye to someone, the viewer, leaving the mill, alternatively he could be greeting a person arriving at the mill.

The windmill in Figure 22 was drawn for the last time in the penultimate session.

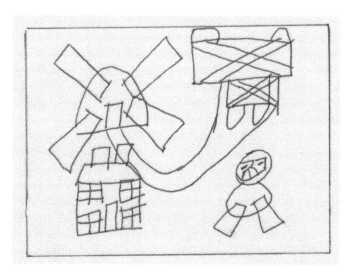

Figure 20 Original Oil pastel on A2 – Windmill (2). Tracing by author.

Positioned at the entrance of the windmill and dominating the whole base of the windmill Edward had drawn a fierce-looking figure with outstretched arms and very enlarged hands. If a welcoming embrace is intended it doesn't look friendly. Maybe the figure which, judging by his hat, is probably a cowboy, is preventing people from entering the windmill. Is this fierce figure positioned inside the mill to keep people out, or are his large hands intended to capture someone?

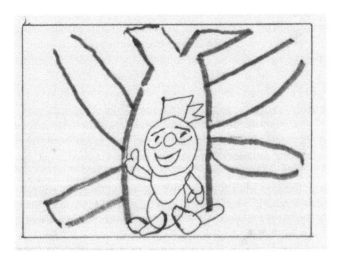

Figure 21 Original – Oil pastel A2 Windmill (3). Tracing by author.

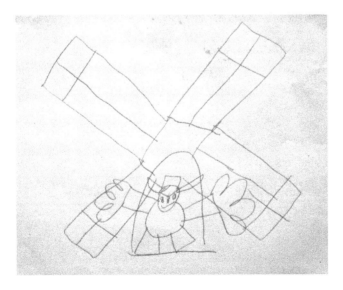

Figure 22 Windmill (4) Pencil A2. Tracing by author.

Iron Man

The 'Iron Man' appeared six months after the start of therapy. He is usually shown as a rectangular figure, whose body consists of two parts; each part can be entered through a door – see Figure 23.

Six months after this first Iron Man a second figure appeared. In this second picture, he smiles and one of the body compartments is without a door. Usually, Iron Man, who gradually began to appear regularly, was drawn alone, and only rarely is he seen with other figures. In the third year, the Iron Man is shown attacking another figure with a claw-like hand, and there was some discussion of protection in this and the previous session. Two months later, when I asked Edward about the compartments of the Iron Man, was it an 'oven or a fridge?', he said 'Frozen Mister'. After two further months the Iron Man is shown with very large hands or claws, and blood coming from his mouth – see Figure 24.

There are no compartments to this version of the Iron Man although there is an additional element placed on top of the head. It seemed important to me to reproduce this drawing in colour in order that the reader should get the full bloody effect.

A week later the Iron Man appears with the compartments restored and teeth at the corners of his mouth. The figure in this picture appears to be stepping out towards the viewer. At the beginning of the third year of therapy, Iron Man is drawn with 'ears that light up' and is, as Edward said, 'sitting down – fallen down'. In the same month Iron Man is wearing a tie that looks like a large penis. When Edward produces his next drawing of the Iron Man he tells me that the top part of the body is a 'wireless' and the bottom part a 'letter box'. This iron man and the next squat

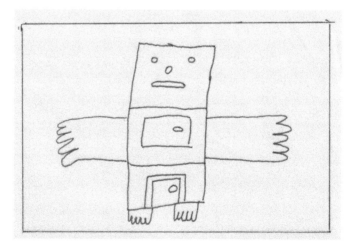

Figure 23 Original Pencil A2 – Iron Man (1). Tracing by author.

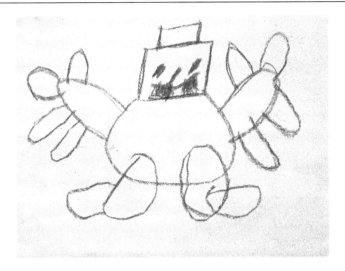

Figure 24 Oil pastel – A2 Iron Man (2).

fat one look less aggressive and Edward suggested that he lights up when 'you press the button'.

In the spring of the fifth year of therapy, Iron Man is drawn pointing a gun at a boy with a cap. A less aggressive looking Iron Man appears in the summer – see Figure 25.

On the far left of this picture is a house and the Iron Man towers above it. He looks surprised (the raised eyebrows) but appears to be smiling. On the far right is drawn a telephone box with a telephone. The Iron Man is connected to the house and the telephone by a wavy line. Edward explained that the Iron Man was speaking to someone in the house.

In this same month, Edward began to use paint and the Iron Man is painted with bold black outline and arms outstretched. We discussed the future at this time and Edward expressed a desire to move to a flat. The Iron Man, however, Edward suggested, 'kicks down flats and buildings'. In the following session, the Iron Man is drawn without arms; instead, Edward reinforces the lines showing legs. Iron Man next appears covered in letters, KE, CD on arms and AB on the bottom section of his body. Edward could not say what the letters were about, except that 'he lights up'. The figure is next shown with a round coat and buttons. The fingers of the Iron Man, in this session, were bitten off by the gorilla. The gorilla was like a lady in the canteen who would not give him a cup of tea and was 'stingy'.

Unusually in November of this year, Iron Man is portrayed by a single round face covering the centre of the paper with an unmistakeably angry mouth. I had just told Edward that I would be away for a week and it did feel as if the human element

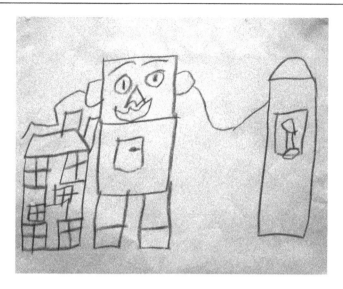

Figure 25 Oil pastel A2 – Iron Man (3).

in the Iron Man's destructiveness could now emerge. Some weeks after this break the Iron Man is shown smiling with arms raised accompanied by the 'king' with a crown. A decorative design of clouds covers the top half of this picture.

In the fifth year of therapy, the Iron Man had a radio in his stomach and lights that lit up. He was run by electricity Edward explained. When I suggested that he looked fierce and probably didn't have any feelings and was not human, but could be switched on and off, he agreed. In the following month, the Iron Man is drawn with a smaller man beside him. The Iron Man 'grinds things up with his teeth, eats things – smashes up the furniture – the mirror' Edward said. After a father Christmas drawing Edward depicted Iron Man standing next to a Christmas tree. This Iron Man also has the characteristic grid-like angry mouth. Iron Man is next shown in pursuit of cars and Edward said 'the iron man crushes the man in the car when he catches him'.

Two months before the end of therapy the Iron Man appears domesticated. He is shown with a farmer and some sheep and Edward said 'the farmer makes sure the Iron Man keeps time'. In the penultimate session Iron Man is shown with a wire connecting one ear to the other across the top of his head – see Figure 26.

This is the last Iron Man picture – Edward again said 'he lights up'. If the line that goes across his head is like the telephone wire then this Iron Man is capable of self-reflection.

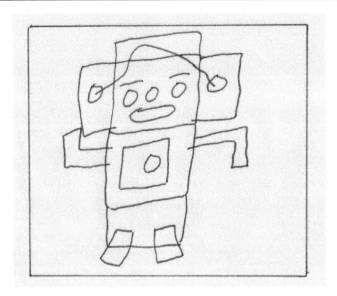

Figure 26 Pencil A2 – Iron Man (4). Tracing by the Author.

Humpty Dumpty

Humpty Dumpty appeared at the end of the first year of therapy. Humpty Dumpty was filled out with colour – see Figure 27.

It is rare for Edward to draw such a complete figure and fill it with colour.

Humpty Dumpty appeared again nine months later and this time is shown 'fallen over', leaning to the right of the picture with a cross around his neck. The ears were prominent but there were no arms to this figure. In the same month, Humpty Dumpty is shown sitting on the wall. In the following month, Humpty Dumpty is shown running after Edward had drawn a man on stilts.

Edward demonstrated that he had some knowledge of the Humpty Dumpty story in the third year of therapy when, he drew a picture of him 'after he's fallen down and broke the bone in his head'. Next month Humpty Dumpty is drawn wearing glasses. At the end of the third year, he draws Humpty Dumpty back sitting on the wall and I asked him about the story. 'He falls mister' he said.

In the Spring of the following year Humpty Dumpty is still drawn on the wall but the next time he appears, in the same month, he is shown as a pirate complete with hat containing a skull and crossbones. The legs of this figure are thick with heavy boots. When Humpty Dumpty next appears, it is through the use of purple paint, sitting on a dark green wall – see Figure 28.

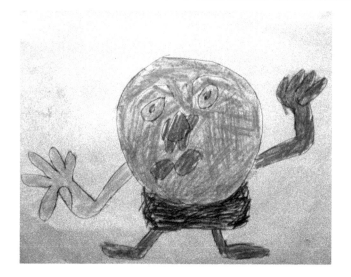

Figure 27 Crayon A2 Humpty Dumpty (1).

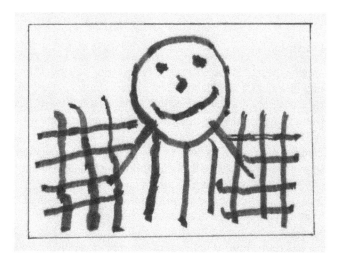

Figure 28 Original Paint on A2 – tracing made by author Humpty Dumpty (2).

Edward explains that he falls down and damages his head but gets it mended. 'Head broke in half', he said. In the following month Humpty Dumpty appears more completely with arms and legs again. In the same session, his parents were drawn, also the Iron Man chasing a car, and the Castle. Humpty Dumpty appears in the last two sessions sitting on the wall smiling.

Couples

As well as single faces or figures, Edward produced many pictures of couples. Usually, the couples were interacting in some way, engaged in a common pursuit, enjoying themselves, or in a competitive relationship, or at cross purposes. The couples began in the sixth month of therapy. They began as two men in a boat, one red and one black, both firing guns – see Figure 29.

These figures firing guns in a boat, unusually, are drawn in profile. The cowboy at the front of the boat has a ring through his nose – maybe he is a pirate of some sort? He also has, what looks like a pigtail?

'Two men in a boat' became the most frequently drawn couple, sometimes rowing together. He did draw a man and woman in a sailing boat together and the image of the sun and the moon continued the male/female theme; the sun having a male face and the crescent moon containing a female figure.

Edward produced several sporting couples, engaged in cricket and football, boxing and wrestling – see Figures 30 and 31.

In Figure 30 which is carefully drawn the ring is superimposed upon the boxers and their genitals are clearly shown under their shorts. Their profile faces seem lumpy and distorted. There is a little circle with a cross in it above the boxer's genitals presumably marking their navels. There also appears to be a corner stool superimposed onto the figure on the right. There is no referee in this drawing or the next picture of Boxers.

In the fourth year of therapy the boxers are shown more abstractly (Figure 31) in this drawing an emphasis is given to the boxing gloves in the centre of the composition where they meet in opposition. Lines appear to represent the ring but also movement and energy.

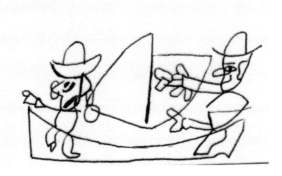

Figure 29 Two Men in a boat. Original Oil Pastel A2 – Tracing made by the author.

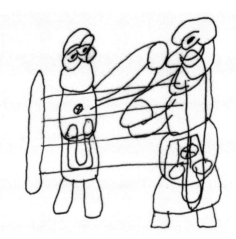

Figure 30 Original Oil Pastel A2 – tracing by the author – Boxers (1).

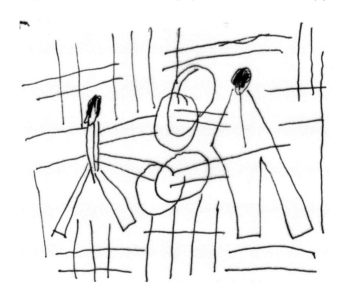

Figure 31 Original Oil Pastel A2 – tracing the author – Boxers (2).

Couples sometimes suffered a common fate. During the second year of therapy, he drew a couple saying 'they're dead in the trees – 1948 War bombed, air raid'. Sometimes the link between us is clearly suggested when, for instance, he shows a couple situated within a rectangular frame, representing the 'cinema' – see Figure 32.

This couple appears in a film. One is bearded, like the therapist. The surrounding rectangle appears in other couple drawings, containing two cowboys, and two figures in a boat.

The two men in a boat became two men in a bath in the third year of therapy – see Figure 33.

One figure is drawn in red crayon and one in black; both figures have round circular bodies with a smaller circle in the centre, presumably a navel, and, as can be seen they are without arms.

This drawing can be compared with Figure 34.

Edward said these were 'boys' in the bath. They seem to be having a good time!

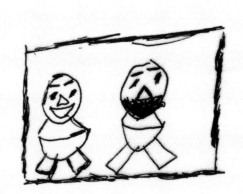

Figure 32 Original Oil Pastel on A2 – cinema tracing by the author.

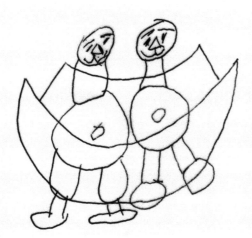

Figure 33 Original Oil Pastel on A2 – 'Two men in a bath' – tracing made by the author.

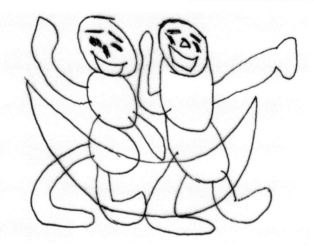

Figure 34 Original Oil Pastel A2 – two boys in bath – tracing by the author.

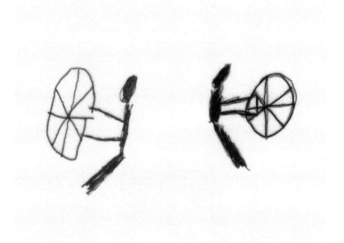

Figure 35 Original Oil Pastel A2 – two 'Drivers' – tracing by the author.

A session was begun with 'two men waiting for a bus' and 'two Chinese waiting for a boat'. Edward had missed a session the previous week and came early but I had asked him to wait. Our Conflicts, difficulties or disagreements, could be represented by a picture of 'two men going round in circles' one of which is given a beard and Edward also drew two men on a see-saw. Simplified red and black figures holding steering wheels show two drivers facing opposite directions – see Figure 35.

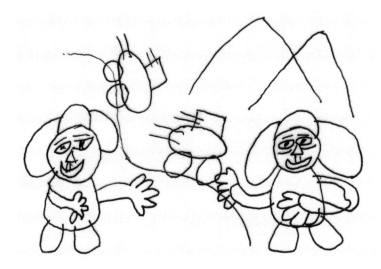

Figure 36 Original Oil Pastel A2 – two judges – tracing by the author.

Another picture shows a doctor on a boat which contains a skeleton. 'The doctor is frightened by the skeleton', Edward explained. Couples could be represented by inanimate objects, two tanks with two clouds above, for example.

Here Edward has drawn two judges, their headgear indicating identity, they stand in front of two tanks battling in two mountains (Figure 36). My thinking is that the judges are engaged in conflict resolution. The line below the mountains rising to the top left, which can be read as two hills, acts like a boarder separating the couple whose gestures towards the tanks and facial expression suggest an appeal to the viewer, to a third beyond the dyad.

The 'Frenchman' and the 'Clown' appear in another couple picture, and in another picture, there are two guards of identical design – see Figure 37.

This made me think of the silence in the sessions.

A couple is shown in another drawing sailing a boat, one man at the bows of the boat and a boy, steering – see Figure 38.

Underneath or surfacing near to this boat is drawn a 'whale'. The man at the front of the boat looks excited to see the whale. One month before the end of therapy, in a cruder drawing, a couple in a boat is shown transporting some 'gold' – 'they're taking it up the river to a factory', Edward said. There are guns on this boat.

These two wrestlers were drawn in the last session, one superimposed upon the other (Figure 39). The smaller one appears to be falling backwards while the larger one leans forward. They have no arms but have round eyes looking directly out at the viewer.

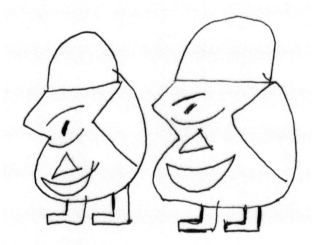

Figure 37 Original Oil Pastel A2 – 'Two Guards – silent ones' – tracing by the author.

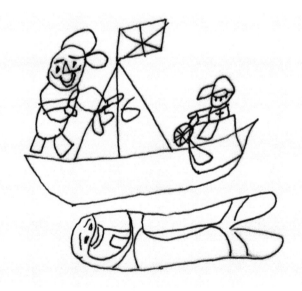

Figure 38 Original Oil Pastel A2 – man, boy and whale – tracing by the author.

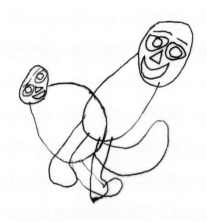

Figure 39 Original Oil Pastel A2 – two wrestlers – tracing by the author.

Reflection and Summary

We can see from the illustrations that I have provided that Edward was able to use his personal visual semiotic to create imaginary figures which were capable of indicating narrative content – we could say, to create a world. Wollheim (1984) in 'The Thread of Life' provides a philosophical account of the mind that is sympathetic to psychoanalysis of the Kleinian kind. He identifies 'iconicity' as a property of some mental states. 'Iconicity' is 'visualizing' and visualizing is 'imagining'. Wollheim writes, 'we should not think that we have to observe our images before we can know what they are... nor that we have to decide what our images mean before we can know what they are of'. In relation to Edward's drawing processes, we could say that in using his repertoire of forms he could surprise himself and discover what they are of as he reaches towards meaning. Wollheim stresses that 'Images' do not 'have to be as determinate as experience' (Wollheim 1984, p63). Through iconic mental states events are imagined. Events contain persons and sequences, and Wollheim suggests that describing the mind as a theatre is helpful to the appreciation of these mental states which involve the imagination and visualizing.

In Wollheim's theatre, there is a dramatist who 'makes up actions' for characters, but he must 'first make up the characters themselves' (p65). Actions, he suggests, can be 'modelled on prototypes' and the nature of the character can place a constraint on actions. 'A character may take time to acquire its consequences' (p66). As well as a dramatist the theatre requires actors. The actor has to 'represent the character to the greatest benefit of his audience'. An audience can be, first, detached, 'permitting itself no affective response' (p67). Second the audience can be 'sympathetic' according to judgements made in relation to characters and their mental states. Thirdly an audience can be empathic, through the selection of a character, 'a protagonist', with whom it shares feeling, for instance, if the character experiences terror so does the empathic audience. In the case of terror, a sympathetic audience might feel pity, and the detached audience might simply judge the feeling as appropriate in the circumstances.

The description above, Wollheim tells us, which makes use of the theatre as an analogy, is incomplete in relation to the understanding of iconic mental states, since roles (dramatist, actor, audience) are 'finely enmeshed one with another' (p71). And there is a particular distinction between 'mental states that possess a point of view and those which don't' (p71). Iconic mental states that make use of visualizing come with a point of view. This point of view can be '*centred*' or '*acentred*' (emphasis in the original). To centrally imagine an event is to 'imagine one person centrally – the person whom I imagine from the inside, the protagonist – and I imagine all the others peripherally'. To imagine an event acentrally 'I imagine everyone acentrally' (p74 & 75).

I would want to argue that Edwards drawings, supported by his verbal comment, were productive of iconic mental states, they represent a form of imagining that involves him as dramatist, actor and audience. His 'little stories' often have protagonists which would enable him to 'centrally' imagine an event, he can imagine more 'acentrally' when the stage is more crowded, or, for instance, where the focus is on couples.

The castle, and the narrative that emerges over time, may more easily be imagined acentrally since it offers many different possible points of view. In the beginning, there are the soldiers who attack the castle, and then the soldiers on the battlements defending the castle, those inside the castle and those outside. Edward explores possibilities for the castle drama in his imagining of events and characters, for instance, children playing on the castle battlements, a soldier who commands a cease fire, an intruder who is shot. As the story emerges, he may find himself centrally imagining a protagonist. Importantly, centrally imagining involves feeling, a feeling that the intruder must be kept out for instance, as is the case when the man makes his way down a ladder to get to the door to keep an enemy out (see Figure 17). It's possible also that he might feel as the intruder feels, or as the children feel who later play on the battlements.

What we should note is that in elaborating the castle theme through drawing, feeling related to the need for defence, to defend an internal space for instance, or to penetrate a defended space, can be experienced. He can, in time, also approach these imagined places and actions from a detached point of view, and consider the way in which the castle differs from the house or church. Edward then notices that the castle interior contains a man inside stoking up a 'big fire'.

Wollheim suggests that an 'event memory' can have the same iconic structure as iconic imagining. However, 'centrally remembering an event is the standard case of event memory' and 'I am necessarily the protagonist of my event-memories – if that is to say, they have one' (p105). Also when I am the protagonist in an event memory 'I don't assume a repertoire, I slip into it' (p119). See my memory of the uniform inspection in Chapter 3. The same kind of work as a dramatist does not seem to apply to events. Wollheim indicates that there are 'mental states which manifest the entanglement of iconic memory with bona fide imagination' (p119). These mental states can be a source of confusion.

The Windmill first appears as imagined, a desirable place to visit, but a source of danger productive of anxiety, a place where the central protagonist could find himself 'caught up' – see Figure 19. Later the Windmill is presented as a reflection on a good, or happy experience, an event at the 'age of twelve'. It provides 'pop', but later, and more imaginatively, it contains 'gold' which needs protection. The Windmill over time becomes the exemplar of the good experience. But there is the boy who runs away from the Windmill to make his way into the house, an indication that there is something in the Windmill which remains threatening. Here there is a memory of the windmill and some entanglement with the imagination. Edward may have experienced something we would regard as bad in the Windmill. One of the questions we might ask here is – is Edward centrally imagining the boy who runs from the Windmill – does he put himself in the boy's shoes? There is only one protagonist in this Windmill scene which involves the boy running – maybe towards the house but Edward does not say. There is a very minimal 'repertoire', as Wollheim would call it, for this imagined character; this could be explained as Edward having simply slipped into the repertoire of a remembered event.

The Iron Man often appeared alone in the drawings and was usually the central protagonist in the narrative or drama that he generated. There was clearly a defensive aspect to the Iron Man's character, an individual, or maybe more appropriately simply a machine, that lacked feeling. He was violent in the beginning but Edward as dramatist enlarged the Iron Man's repertoire in relation to action and interaction with others, and we can witness a development from dangerous machine towards the emergence of a thinking communicating and feeling being. The Iron man in his later appearances communicates between the telephone and the house, he is disciplined by the farmer who ensures that he 'keeps time', he has wires moving through his head, and he 'lights up'. What was refrigerator becomes electricity and the Iron Man can be switched on and off, and he is finally shown as capable of reflection.

We are naturally inclined to think of Humpty Dumpty as a cultural figure that enables Edward to explore his experiences, feelings and thoughts in relation to Learning Disability. But there is the possibility, and necessity, of making use of other cultural figures in this way, for instance 'Dopey' in 'the seven dwarfs', and 'educating Archie'. Since 'prototypes'… 'can place a constraint' on a characters actions, as Wollheim suggests, then a range of prototypical characters are required to explore complications that the notion of Learning Disabilities covers.

Communication and relating were developed as a theme in the Iron Man pictures, present in the Windmill series and in the stories emerging around the castle. But the drawings of couples seem to involve Edward in thinking about, and imagining relation, in a more focussed way. The couples present a variety of possible relations. The relation of male to female, man and boy, couples sharing adventures, couples in a form of competitive relating, and couples in opposition to each other – not relating, or refusing relationship. Complication was possible in his visualizing of couples who also relate to a third Other, for example Figure 36 of the Two Judges, and the Man, Boy and Whale drawing, Figure 38. Of course it is difficult not to think of the couples as indicating changes in the therapeutic relation, of which, neither Edward or myself, were fully conscious.

Wollheim himself builds his example of iconic imagination on his reading of Gibbon, and imagines himself as Sultan Mohomet II, as he enters Constantinople. The example highlights the philosopher's literary and educational resources, and may well be reflected in the exhaustive and complicated nature of his theatrical model which identifies a range of mental states and dispositions generated through visualizing. Edward's visual imagination displays *his* cultural resources, which reflect a working-class environment, and his cultural consumptions. His imagined characters possess a more limited repertoire of actions, perhaps. Nevertheless, Edward did demonstrate that he was able to develop his thinking about his characters over time, that he was capable of experiencing 'belief, desire, and feeling' (Wollheim 1984, p81) and capable of processing affective and sensory experience through the use of his form of iconic imagination, which may not replicate Wollheim's model in its entirety.

I have linked Edward's drawing to the production of mental states, as Wollheim describes them. Some of Edward's drawings might be assessed as crude, often when used to generate imaginary figures and dramas, but this maybe because his visualizing is spontaneous and rapid, but Edward has demonstrated that drawing, as visualizing and imagining, can have its own particular vivacity. Through its physical presence, and its sensory qualities, its plenitude and semiotic potential, it is able to transcend the sensory impoverishment of verbal imagining, in this respect it is capable of communicating feeling in a particularly vivid way and this, I would argue, is why drawing is important to Edward. Here I will simply refer the reader back to Figures 13 and 14.

I would now wish to end this exploration of Edward's use of the available art materials and note that Edward's drawing was produced in the context of a developing therapeutic relationship, a relationship that emerges in a particular setting, and it would now seem important to attempt to provide some account of that context, so that we can approach his work from a fresh vantage point.

PART 3

Narrative and Reflection

Bion points out that reports are not 'exempted from our own findings', that memory 'should not be treated as more than a pictorialized communication of an emotional experience', that the narratives he provided should be regarded as fictions, and the expectation that 'the record represents what actually took place must be dismissed as vain' (Bion 1967, p1, p2 and p120). Bion's position stresses the partiality of reports, they are reports made by somebody, about someone else, and about a shared situation. Reports are also about the fiction that a report can give an objective account of events.

I have tried to be honest in my construction of this therapeutic narrative but I am conscious of the inadequacy of my note-taking and I am aware of the possibility of unconscious phantasies and repressions promoting distortions, that inevitably creep in unnoticed, adding a fictional element to my story. Nevertheless I am hopeful that *something* of the original emotional experience of working with Edward will be transmitted in the following account of the therapeutic journey.

The narrative I present below is based upon my note-taking completed after each session. What notes I have used I have edited since in many sessions very little passed between Edward and myself in terms of words and a listing of the images produced quickly becomes tedious. I have therefore tried to focus on the images that seem to me to be important at the time, but I have also tried to impart some sense of the repetitive, nature of some of Edward's drawing activity. Reflection contemporary with the writing and editing for this publication has been added and appears in italics.

Year 1

April

Edward arrived at the department with a nurse. He was a short man, a little over five foot tall, a slim figure giving the impression of being strong and healthy. He was well turned out in a tweed sports jacket, looking like an enthusiastic jockey. Edward gave very little eye contact. He smiled quite a lot, sometimes his smile became a grin, sometimes, more fleetingly, it became something close to a painful grimace. Edward did not use much gesture and since his facial expressions were limited it was difficult to make a judgement in relation to his feelings.

In this first session, he drew a house with palm trees using crayons. I asked him if it is in a hot country and he replied 'Switzerland'. His next picture seemed more ambitious and he named the subject as he proceeded – 'River, a bridge, speed boat, ship going into the harbour'. This was followed by another bridge over the 'River Thames'. A castle was drawn with 'a man playing a drum'. There were sentries on the battlements, plus three other figures, two inside the castle. He drew a man with a pipe and seemed pleased with the result. Two heads came next, one named a 'cowboy'. Edward also made a house from coloured paper which was cut into rectangles and stuck down confidently.

A ship reaching harbour, the castle and the house, suggested to me an arrival, perhaps a feeling of reaching home, and the bridges seemed hopeful. The drummer, however, was perhaps alerting the castle occupants of some future danger.

I kept these associations to myself and I noted that Edward had used the art materials enthusiastically. He seemed to want to impress me with his skills. He did name items that he had drawn, and he identified actions ('man playing a drum'). I did think his responses to my questions were limited, but I felt that the session indicated that Edward had an ability to use the art materials with communicative intent.

I gave him a cup of tea in this first session, as he asked for a drink. This was in keeping with the culture of the institution as patients expected a drink whenever they attended any of the hospital departments. I realise, of course that the tea, represented something more than simple refreshment, but I did hope that we had, in this setting, begun to establish a form of exchange, where I would provide materials and a quiet space in which he could work, and in which we could together explore the imagery that emerged.

Following this start, which I felt was promising, attendance quickly became intermittent and brief, when we did meet, the meetings lasted for 15 minutes, sometimes more, sometimes less. These were meetings that seemed to be filled with anxiety. Edward would draw very rapidly for a few minutes, then quickly retreat, saying 'I'm going now mister' while avoiding eye contact, and, more significantly, avoiding my comments, questions or any kind of speech.

I did think that I had given him some explanation in relation to the referral and Art Therapy, but I did not know what his understanding was, or exactly what his wishes were in relation to the offer of the space, the use of the materials, and my attention and support, except through his actions. When I asked him if he wanted to come, during the sessions he responded with 'yes mister – yes mister' but when seen outside of the department after missing sessions he said 'no mister'.

During the summer months, there were prolonged absences and I began to feel that Edward's anxiety and ambivalence, which seemed to centre mostly around my speech and encouragement of speech, were likely to end my attempts at providing therapy. He was consistent in avoiding any prolonged verbal interaction with me.

The sessions were scheduled for 2.30 p.m. I learnt from the ward staff that Edward often simply wandered off in the morning after eating his breakfast, and nobody would be quite sure where he was, at any particular time. He did occasionally call in to departments in the hope of gaining cigarettes, and he usually returned to the ward for meals. I then made an agreement with the ward staff that we should change the time for therapy sessions from afternoons to first thing in the morning, and that Edward should be regularly escorted. This disciplinary intervention, which placed me in a position of authority, in alignment with the ward staff, seemed to pay off, and Edward, in October began to settle down to a more consistent attendance. He established a pattern of using the oil pastels and paper greedily, working his way through several boxes of pastels which, when they broke, which they always did because he drew in a very energetic, forceful and hurried manner, were cast aside. As he usually left abruptly, the broken pastels and crayons lay scattered across the table next to a pile of paper, 30 sheets or more, containing his drawings, at the end of the session. In the new year, he began to make his way to sessions independently and be regular in his time keeping. He maintained control in relation to the ending of the session, in this way holding on to some autonomy and challenging my power.

Year 2 (First Full Year)

February

On arrival, Edward speaks as he begins his first drawing – 'Do some drawing Mister'. He placed the first drawing between us. Edward said, 'An owl – they look like that'.

I was thinking that the owl looked cubist and said – 'You have an unusual style of drawing Edward'. He responded, 'Yes style mister'. Next he drew a windmill and he says that he saw a film of a windmill where 'a man gets inside it starts working and goes round and round – he gets caught up'.

After this, he busily works at a pattern and asks 'where's that cup of tea mister?' I make him tea. Contained in the shapes of his pattern are a horse, an owl, swastikas, anchors and a bottle. Other shapes appear and he tells me that a policeman is going to Buckingham Palace to get some change – not the changing of the guards 'money' he says. Next he does a drawing of 'custard man' – 'he lives in a den'. I asked about the face of custard man, 'is he smiling?' he does not respond to the question but quickly moves on to the next drawing of an 'Indian'. I linked this Indian to a drawing of an Indian made in the previous session, who was 'looking round the house'. Edward then asks for another cup of tea. I respond with – 'only one'. He draws 'an old woman – not a witch'. He ends his drawing with 'a teacher'.

I asked Edward to look through the pictures with me, and I pointed out that it seemed difficult to look, as he was on the point of leaving. I gave a brief account of the things he *had* said and I suggested that we didn't know what those things were about yet. This was met with silence and I asked if he thought of me as 'a teacher'. 'No mister' was his answer. The silence leaves me frustrated, but whatever Edward had thought, or felt, in relation to my comment, he was clearly indicating that he had said enough, as he began leaving as I spoke.

Now that he was coming regularly and seemed more committed to the process of making drawings and showing them to me, albeit briefly, I had the idea that he felt that since he had entered into the Art Therapy department he was caught up in some kind of machine, trapped in a relationship. 'Custard man' cannot be discussed. It is worth noticing that when I suggest, somewhat lamely, that 'we' didn't know what 'those things were about yet'. The word 'yet' implies that 'we' (the hospital, myself, and possibly Edward?) will know in time. It maybe that Edward had felt that he had given a sufficient account of what the drawings were about. But my speech here takes the form of an implied demand, a demand for a verbal confession, that will be realised in time, that Edward would give a full account of himself. I felt obliged, using my Kleinian frame, to think that the 'old woman – who is 'not a witch', but I feel obviously is, and the 'teacher', must relate to the therapist who refuses to give extra tea, but one who also applies pressure in relation to speech. If Edward has demands for tea I have unwelcome, sinister, and covert, demands of my own.

May

Edward arrived early but was allowed to wait in the speech therapy department next door and the Speech Therapist provided him with coffee. At the beginning, there was a moment of sharpening pencils together which, for me, felt hopeful. Unusually he took some initiative in conversation and asked for help. The pencils were put aside ready for use.

He began by drawing faces. He was willing to give most of the faces titles. There was a striking face which I assumed from the hat must be a pirate. He then called my attention to – 'Them ships Mister'. I drew his attention to the skull and cross bones on the hat (see Figure 14). 'I didn't do that mister – it was there already' he said. I suggested that he couldn't talk about this image and did not want to be connected to it. This was followed by a 'teacher' and 'a pig'. The pig was followed by a 'little piggy'. He asked for more coffee and I then began to amuse myself by wondering if he was not, after all, a little piggy. One face had teeth in a grid form suggesting anger but Edward did not want to say anything about this when I pointed to the teeth.

He next drew a 'gypsy man – on a donkey' – 'the ones you see with donkeys mister'. This man had a toothy grin.

I felt the need to make some sort of comment, a summary at this point. Edward saw that I was about to speak and immediately responded with – 'I'm going now mister' – before I could say anything. He was soon outside the door and I was left feeling enraged – rendered useless. It felt very personal. In that moment, I decided to go after him and called him back saying – 'I've got something to say before you go – take a seat'. He surprised me and came back inside and took a seat. Leafing through the drawings I suggested to him that maybe he felt like a little piggy today asking for more coffee and that I was like the teacher, telling him to come back inside and sit down. He looked down at the drawings, his face taking on a serious expression, chastised but seemingly listening.

We can see that in this session the theme of Edward's hunger, a call for more coffee, and his difficulty, or refusal, in relation to speech, present in February, two months previous, is given further development. My 'take a seat' is a command in the form of a demand for reciprocity, but it is also disciplinary and reinforces the power relation embedded in the institutional setting. It seems that I must have my comment and summary heard in silence – just as the 'teacher' might demand obedience from the 'little piggy'. How is the 'enraged' feeling generated? I would argue it is in the angry mouth and toothy grin of the 'gypsy man' as well as the abrupt attempt at departure as soon as I begin to speak. I am also aware that Edward is going to leave lots of broken pastels scattered across the table. I am then left in pieces.

If Edward's attempt at a rapid exit is regarded as Edward's desire to evacuate his aggressive contemptuous self, leave his destruction, the scattered pieces of his world inside the therapist, what do the pictures and Edward's actions achieve for him? It encourages the therapist to 'act out' in relation to his, the therapist's, frustrations, but maybe in a way which provides some containment. These exchanges might be regarded as exemplifying, in this context, infantile phantasies related to the transference and countertransference. The hunger on my part is for some form of validation, or recognition that I might have something to offer.

I did think that Edward's comment in relation to the skull and crossbones represented a denial, but maybe we should think about it as a need for Edward to distance himself from the image of death, which after all is, in a hallucinatory sense, 'already' 'there', awaiting both of us, as Edward contemplates the image in response to my inquiry.

July

Edward began drawing while looking at the work of others on the wall. He described the figures he produced in response as 'comic cuts'. He held on to the activity of drawing until the end of the session, thus avoiding talk. He did, however, label his drawings. There was a German plane bombing a ship, a 'snow man and snow boy – me'. There were two versions of this and the second version seemed to contain bits inside the figures – maybe genitals? A house without windows. I asked what it might be like inside – 'don't know mister'. A later house has ghosts in the window. The 'iron man' and 'Humpty Dumpty' appear next and the session ends with a drawing of a cat. As he had been coming early and finding that I was not here I emphasised the starting time for the following week.

This session was typical of many sessions during this second year, in that they were often passed in silence, apart from the sound of his drawing, and the labelling of imagery.

October (1)

Arrived at 9.05 a.m. and began drawing animals using pencils but colouring in the body with crayons. I suggested to him that he could use paint but he said that he liked crayons and didn't use paint. Was he telling me not to interfere? The first animal something… 'us'. This was repeated but Edward could not articulate the word and in the end decided he would call it a 'donkey'. Maybe it was a hippopotamus. The second animal was an elephant, next a pig, then a bull. All were coloured. I encouraged him to say more about the animals but he did not go beyond labelling them and agreeing with whatever I said, e.g. I said 'big bull' – 'That's right mister – big bull' he replied. A face coloured in green followed this was labelled as 'a boy'. 'Humpty Dumpty' and two people rowing in a boat came next. I suggested that it could be us on a journey, rowing. I also remarked that things were filled out with colour today, as if they were more real. He worked past the 10.00 a.m. ending and was reluctant to leave.

Edward was engaged in some play, which, to some degree, constituted a personal and private process and space, from which I felt excluded. He did want more time in this session to generate more imagery.

October (2)

Edward came after I telephoned the ward at 9.10 a.m. The cleaners were around in the department and I was in the office and the cleaners alerted me to Edward's presence after he had begun work in the studio. After he had been drawing for about 15 minutes a nurse then arrived to say that he has to go to the dentist. He left with the nurse and came back in ten minutes – 'I told you I wouldn't be long didn't I'. He said that he would do three more drawings then go.

Surprisingly he asked me to look through the drawings and I pointed to the large ears on the faces and said how they 'the cowboys' must be listening – paying attention, using their senses. I compared this to the clown who had no ears. However, the next clown that appeared in the pile of drawings did have large ears, and he pointed this out. He then talked about clowns quite spontaneously and freely: how they did magic tricks; how they climbed ladders and poured down buckets of water. There were two clowns on one sheet, with different hats, apart from the hats they looked identical. After the clowns came a policeman. I said that he looked serious and I asked if he was going to arrest the clowns. There was a third clown that followed – 'looks like a lemon' he said – 'I'll call that one lemon clown'. He then talked about clowns in the street and related that – 'In the old days when there were trams about people all came out of doors to have a look'.

*He does manage to work, or play, with or without me, entertaining himself with clowns and his reminiscences about the 'old days'. He was demonstrating more confidence in the setting and there was spontaneous conversation. The cowboys were using their ears and this reflects his listening to me, perhaps, but also my **not** listening out for him while I am in the office, and not opening my door to have a look. My retreat to the office while waiting for him is a response to feeling redundant, and the clowns reflect the comedy of our relationship.*

November

Edward was having some blood taken from him so we started late at 9.30 a.m. but ended at 10.15 a.m. He began rapidly producing faces which changed from face to face as he progressed through his pile of paper. Faces with tongues out changed to something more fearsome. When we were both looking at the drawings I pointed to the tongue growing larger and asked him if it was the clown who played card tricks and poured water from ladders, as he had added a clown's hat. He said it was cowboys but then followed with a hat which he agreed was the teacher's hat. I said how the feeling seemed to change from a cheeky clown who played tricks to an angry face with large teeth. The faces ended with a woman whose face was 'like a pig', and I suggested that the drawings showed how his mood was changing. In response to my comments, he repeated 'Yes mister', but he appeared to be listening and he did not want to avoid looking at the pictures.

A relationship was established in this second year during which Edward grew in confidence and was willing to initiate speech, mostly in the form of naming items the characters or items he had drawn, and at times he was willing to listen to my interpretative comment. I was required to learn to respect the silence and to contain my frustration.

Year 3

January

Drawings began with fountains and a bridge. There were cowboys on a boat with an aeroplane overhead. In the boat were large phallic-looking faces that Edward said were 'bombs'. The bombs belonged to the cowboys rather than the aeroplane. Two stage coaches, on one a 'cowboy-bandit' who, Edward explained, jumps off the stage coach onto people, killing them. The windmill appeared and Edward said that the cowboy nearby was guarding against robbers who robbed gold from the dungeon underneath the windmill. A cat was stealing milk from a milk-cart. Edward said that 'cats bite you'. As we were looking through the pictures I was, as usual, trying to find a way of summarising the themes but found it difficult to make sense of it all. Not unusually, Edward gave the impression of not wanting to hear from me and left promptly at 10.00 a.m.

Later using my Kleinian frame I reflect on the aggressive phantasies of dropping bombs, phallic and anal, except the bombs with faces in the boat do not quite fit this frame. I was thinking that there is a need to defend the good, the gold in the windmill. Related to this I also noticed the orally aggressive cat that steals the milk.

February

He produced 30 or so cowboy faces. The first face had a tongue out. Their hats changed colour but apart from the change of colour and the disappearing tongue the smile on the face remained. As he was grinning and smiling a lot, I pointed to the tongue and suggested that it was cheeky and maybe this was how he felt this morning. He said that the cowboys were Kit Carson, Roy Rogers and Billy the Kid. The succession of cowboys blocked my thinking and Edward's fixed facial expression suggested defiance of a kind. I suggested to him that we might look at the previous week's drawing, hoping that this would generate some thinking related to the cowboys. But he did not respond to my prompt and left ten minutes before the end.

For whatever reason, Edward wanted to remain hidden behind his cowboy masks, and he asserted his independence by leaving early. The confidence in relating to me in a spontaneous way, present at the end of year 2, seemed to be disappearing.

April

He began by looking through the crayons and he emptied out a tub, searching for a particular colour. He started his drawing with a helicopter, which was followed by figures. I remarked how the figures had no arms or legs and they were strange. Edward laughed and I pointed out that the legs, if they had any, looked like penises. He continued to laugh then drew his hand and then mine. When drawing he glanced at his hand and he also showed me a cut on his finger. He said that he didn't know how he got it. I showed concern by looking closely at his finger. There seemed to be an intimate contact of a kind taking place, and there was some eroticism involved in this exchange around the fingers and hands which follow on from the penises.

The hands were followed by a boat with an engine, and a letterbox. When asked, he said that he did not receive letters or write any, but he would like to receive letters. A stagecoach without wheels leads me to remark on the lack of wheels. Edward said it was alright but I then pointed out that he was not looking, he then looked and changed the drawing, adding wheels. I suggested to him that he maybe thought that I did not look at the pictures or think about them, and maybe it was hard for him to think about them. Two 'Chineses rowing a boat' followed this exchange. There was also a ship on the river Thames – 'People inside going away', he said.

He drew two men between trees and said – 'They're dead in the trees, 1948 war, bombed air raid' '– he used to listen to the air raid 'when in pram' he explained. I asked if frightening – 'Yes mister'. A cowboy face he calls 'monk'. The word 'monk' made me think of total institutions and abstinence. I said that maybe he, the monk, lives in an institution, alone, and doesn't have any girls (I was thinking of the eroticism of the earlier part of the session). He wanted to leave early but I asked him to stay and he produced two cowboys with guns. I suggested that the two dead people could be us and maybe it was frightening to look at pictures about the air raids.

I am not sure why I should think that the two dead people might be us, and the mention of 'girls' was not helpful. Maybe I was fearful of something dying in the relationship, if we could not communicate spontaneously. The desire for letters did suggest to me, a wish to participate in symbolic exchanges and that I should not give up on speaking, questioning, and inevitably, interpreting. When I made more direct comments on the drawings, the lack of wheels on the stagecoach seemed to bring us closer together again.

June (1)

Edward came on time. There were lots of guns in this session: two men on a boat with guns and two men on a lorry with guns. One man on 'lorry', initially labelled 'speedboat', also with gun. Two men on church roof with guns. He did not want to stop drawing to look at work or give further comment. When I comment on there being little time to think about the meaning he replies with the usual 'yes mister'. I point out all the guns. He tells me that a man with a gun goes into the house. I ask who is he going to shoot – 'Nobody he's putting the gun in a drawer'.

He asks if he can go now and I point out that there is five minutes left and he draws a castle which has men with guns on the battlements. I suggest to him that he places his violent angry bit away in a drawer and now he needs a castle to protect himself, 'for protection' – 'to be safe'. I suggest that he might think that I had a gun. He said 'Yes protection mister'. He ends with a flag on the castle.

His enemy or enemies are not identified but he is sure that he needs protection. Asking if he can go suggests he is willing to give way to me. When he leaves I am left wondering about paranoid phantasies. The institution generates paranoia, and he naturally wants to protect himself against staff.

July

Following a holiday he arrived late and I was in the office but he did not let me know that he had arrived and sat- down and began drawing. I suggested to him that he was telling me that he could get on well enough without me, and that he had managed through the holiday on his own. While he was drinking tea I asked if we could look through the drawings. 'Yes mister OK' he said but then he appeared to want to go on drawing without stopping. I intervened by removing some paper and I said that it was important that we look and try to think about the drawings. Edward responded angrily, perhaps the most articulate I've ever known him to be, he said 'Don't interfere – I'll stop doing it – didn't you know that's what happens if you interfere – I'll stop doing it'. I said that I realised it was difficult to think about the drawings but I suggested he could try.

A ship with funnels and wheels follows – 'sinking mister – ship' he said. A stagecoach with three cowboys, grid-like teeth, which I pointed to, followed by an aeroplane and a train. A house, trees and cloud over head came next. I asked about the clouds, 'good sign, or bad sign?' – 'A bad sign – a bad sign mister' he said.

Next came 'faces in the sky mister' smiling, and a figure he named 'the Devil'. Faces then followed, firstly smiling, then with the grid-like mouth and smile together, one mouth on top of the other. These faces were followed by one face smiling, and three faces with the grid-like mouth, which indicates anger. I suggested to him that he may be struggling to join together parts of his mind, the bad 'devil' angry part, and the good smiling happy part, and that it may be very difficult to know what to do with the angry bit. Two figures with a rocket in between followed and I then pointed to the rocket and suggested that this could happen in here if 'the angry bit got in here – it would be like a rocket going up'. Finally alternate faces were drawn, a smiling face, an angry face, then a face with a confused mouth, then an angry face again.

I gave some paper back and I said that I realised that one of the things he valued, was 'not being interfered with' – 'me not interfering with the drawing'. He said that the two figures he drew next were 'in the forest in the snow, it was cold'. I suggested that he maybe thought I was cold towards him sometimes, going on holiday and 'not thinking about him in the office – not noticing him come in'.

The sinking ship appears after my interference, suggesting that there may be some danger to the relationship, through my insistence on limits in relation to the amount of material available, and the demand for some speech, in particular that demand for something in relation to the drawings. But I do seem to have come back from the holiday determined to offer Edward my interpretative comments, which are not always helpful. Edward through his faces does appear to be struggling with his feelings, bringing together good and bad feeling, which was much more palpable in this session. Maybe Edward was thinking, could he risk being angry, by saying what he thinks? He did at the beginning and was consequently very articulate. While I make a demand for reflection, Edward seeks to limit the influence of the 'devil'. He might, of course, regard me as the devil when I provocatively interfere.

Year 4

February (1)

A difficult start. Edward was five minutes late and after he arrived, I realise that I need to fetch him some paper from another room. But I also answer a telephone call which I feel I am obliged to answer as the answer phone is not on. I apologised to Edward and tell him that I will add five minutes to the end to allow for the telephone call.

While I am fetching the paper and answering the telephone he draws two people, a boat and fire engine. He draws 'the badge of the Royal Artillery' containing a tiger and gun. I asked him if he knew anybody in the Royal Artillery. He says 'no' and I suggest that it's a badge to show how brave and fierce a person can be, and I suggest that maybe it is a warning to me about him. Three men – French men (with hats) on hills. Next the judge Edward said – 'In court'. The Iron Man and two boys. The iron man has a tie which looks to me very like a penis and I say to Edward maybe this is a powerful father, with a big penis, who is cold and hard towards boys. He listens. Next a man with a pipe and two boys playing cricket. Cowboy and Humpty Dumpty – before he has fallen off his wall I suggest. This is followed by a man 'running late for a bus'. I pointed out that he was late this morning. A thatched cottage comes next and Edward points to the 'Hay', there is a boy inside and a man outside, the boy has a mouth turned down whereas the man is smiling. I then spoke about my being outside on the phone when he's in here and I ask him how that feels. Edward then draws a windmill and house and he tells me that he prefers to live in a windmill (after I ask). Next is drawn, two men one 'Churchill – the old bugger' he also has a tie/penis. I remark on *somebody* being tough, having a big penis, and I suggest that maybe he is wondering which one of us is tough. Charlie Chaplin follows Churchill and I say how he is a softer and different kind of person, a clown who is sad. Edward agrees with sad. Maybe you are wondering what kind of person you are. Are you 'a tough bugger Churchill' or a Charlie Chaplin – softer person, or sad clown. He next draws a boy with big eyes 'looking'. I say how he looks surprised or shocked, 'I wonder what he has seen?' I suggest that we use our eyes 'here', looking at pictures and drawing. He draws a cinema, two people outside 'waiting to get in', followed by two men sitting down 'on screen'. I linked this to the session, the time boundary and start, and suggested that maybe he was telling me about the importance of 'starting and finishing on time'. Next, he draws a man sitting down 'reading a newspaper', a 'prince standing' with large tie. This important man, the 'prince', is being ignored, I suggest, Edward agreed, 'Yes he's ignoring him'. I linked this to his being ignored this morning. Just at this moment, we were then disturbed by another patient who had arrived early for her session. I take her outside and she is laughing madly. We quickly look at the last few pictures together, they include 'Men on the main road', a car, 'houses by the fields', and a cowboy.

*Edward was, I think, in this session, willing to listen to my comments and suggestions, but he was also telling me to behave properly, keep good time, like the judge 'in court' perhaps, and remain attentive. I do seem to be gratifying **my** needs in this session, answering the telephone call, and giving lots of suspect interpretative comments, but at least he seemed to listen and his drawings do suggest he is making something from my interpretative comments. The main road makes me think of Edward on the motorway, the adventure that led to him being referred to Art Therapy.*

May

Edward missed the previous session as he was taken out on a trip to visit a community facility. He came early and asked for a session on the previous day; he came early again on this day, the day of his session. Some people playing football, two playing cricket, two men waiting for a bus. I linked the waiting for a bus to him missing a session the previous week. He said that he wanted to come. Two 'Chinese waiting for their boat', followed by tanks. Windmill – 'it's the windmill by the forest – is it still there?' he asks. He thinks it is, and says, 'you can get pop there' 'From the windmill?' I ask – 'yes 7pence a bottle'. 'Olden time truck' follows 'carrying jumble – tips up the jumble – you know in the olden times' I ask what sort of jumble – 'Oh stores and things'. I said how maybe in the olden times here in the past your mind was filled with jumble but now you are able to think a bit more clearly – 'you've tipped some of it out'. 'No' he responded in an emphatic fashion.

He next drew the Iron man and I asked what was inside the doors – 'top one wireless bottom one letter box'. I said he seemed like a robot – 'you give him a message and he does what you ask – carries out the orders'. 'That's right mister'. 'Maybe this is how you feel in here?' Two cars on the road 'going in different directions' are drawn. Also on the same theme, two drivers back to back with steering wheels. I point out how the drivers are going in opposite directions. Two boxers follow, then an aeroplane and bombs, and a large tank with people. A large cannon with smoke is drawn, Edward says, 'gun fired'. I spoke about the sport theme and suggested maybe he felt we were having a competition, a competition to decide what time we were going to start.

Edward is given messages and he operates like the robotic iron man. When Edward asks about the windmill, – 'is it still there?'. In coming the day before, and in coming early, is he checking to see that the Art Therapy department is still there?

*Maybe this is the real question. My interpretation in relation to the 'jumble' is wishful thinking and a complete **waste** of time. Edward is quite sure that he has not tipped any jumble out. It's good to know that he can reject my comments. Maybe his thinking has gained in clarity but he points out that we are sometimes driving in opposite directions. Or we are in competition with one another. His bombs, and the large tank, and a large gun could represent a development of the ritualised violence of the boxers. He is aware of our differences, and we are both struggling to reconnect after the missed session. Why didn't I offer him an extra session as he was going on a community visit? Maybe I didn't have enough notice. The images of the Windmill, the Iron Man and the boxers, the drivers going in an opposite direction all represent aspects of our relationship.*

June

Going slow in the beginning and willing to talk about each picture in turn. This is a recent development I thought. First, he draws 'Mexico and dunce' he explained that 'dunce had trouble with his head – couldn't make his legs walk'. I said maybe you had trouble with your head sometimes and were unable to do the things you wanted to do. 'Yes, Yes' he said, with a clear note of irritation. This was followed by a difficult silence.

The next picture was of a cowboy with large gun; the paper positioned in such a way that the gun points towards me. I was thinking about this picture in relation to the way that his, 'Yes, yes' appeared abrupt and was aimed at ending the exchange around 'trouble' with heads, and I then suggested that he might be angry about his difficulties and felt people didn't understand, 'went too quickly'. 'No' he responded. This was also delivered in an abrupt way. A baby smiling in the pram, bike and boy. The boy owned the bike, he did not have one when little he told me. A man 'lemon-head – there used to be lemon-heads in the hospital'. I said how we had a happy baby, then a boy, and then a man who had not turned out right – 'something happened'. He drew next a man with 'two horns' – 'the horns affected his head made him forget things and he lost his medal'. I asked if he forgot things – 'sometimes, yes'. Gorilla next and then he ended his session with 'Devil in the sky', 'with horns' and 'medals'. After the session, I began thinking that maybe it is the devil in him that affects his thinking. Before his mention of the dunce I was wondering about his 'handicap' (whatever that might be), and what does the medal indicate?

I responded to the dunce subject stupidly, in an over-enthusiastic way. In retrospect I think that people going 'too quickly' is less of a problem for Edward than people, the therapist in particular, not appreciating that there maybe all sorts of feelings entailed in having trouble with your head. Maybe the gun, which made me think of anger, was simply defensive in response to the pain experienced in discussing and acknowledging his difficulties and losses and I should have shown more sensitivity in relation to this pain. 'Lemon head' is a reference to residents in the hospital who have dysmorphic features. The devil with his horns seems to be linked to this group. Losing the medal does indicate losing something important and it could be that Edward not having a bicycle when a small boy was significant in relation to the notion of handicap.

September

Following the summer break, Edward came on time. He was smiling. I said welcome back, and he responded 'Yes, Yes'. I thought – well he *seemed* to be pleased to be back.

He drew two cowboys with 'telephone thing in between them', followed by more couples, cowboys, boys playing, two prisoners, boys and prisoners given names – 'Peter, Geoffrey, Morgan and Allen'. These are names he has mentioned before and I think that they refer to other male hospital residents he knows. Two women are drawn next, one with 'bear fur around her' – 'stuck up' he said. The 'other one wasn't'. Both women were 'crying'. Then Humpty Dumpty 'after he fell down' – 'Broken the bone in his head'. I asked if the women were crying because of the accident to Humpty. 'Could be' he said.

The donkey man came next – 'the donkey man – rides across the desert on donkey' he told me. Then a sailor – 'sails goes on the sea'. He draws a boat tied up, moored against a quay, and then a picture of the 'captain'. I linked these drawings to my coming back after the holidays. These drawings were followed with the iron man who has lights and is square-looking. 'When you press buttons he lights up' Edward said. I suggested this was the warm feeling he had at the beginning. The Iron man is followed by a 'fire engine' then the last picture an engine that 'goes along the bottom of the sea' it has a 'black man inside'. I did feel later that this was a positive return to work, work which is creative, which is also play.

Edward was using his capacities to generate images which were related to suggestive beginnings, or maybe the ending of stories. The last picture with its submarine theme could be interpreted as containing repressed, unconscious or unexpressed, feelings about the holidays. Year 4 is about negotiating differences and my learning sensitivity in relation to his communications which are often present in a sequential form in the imagery.

Year 5

January

Indians were drawn on the first sheet of paper which he places in front of himself so that I could see. He described them as 'different sort of Indians – a chief – he goes into the tent and burns himself in the fire puts his hand in and tries to light a cigarette'. Cowboys and Charlie Chaplin follow, next a man who 'has broken bone in his head – goes to the hospital to get it mended, doesn't speak but reads the newspaper – the star or standard – his head on a pillow'. I ask Edward if he knows why he came into the hospital – 'No'. Then he tells me that his dad is in the hospital now – 'sits in a chair – he's old now – doesn't come to see me anymore'. Do you miss him I ask – 'yes' – would you like to visit him in hospital – 'Yes' he says but no more. This is followed with a face that he names 'coco', then 'some blokes' and a full figure in profile with crosses, he says 'a vicar – clergyman' and this is followed by some more Indians.

I passed on his comment about visiting his father to the ward staff but a visit was not arranged and I later regret not following it up with the ward. The man in the hospital reading the newspaper is likely to be his Father who now is unable to speak. The clergyman suggested to me an imminent death.

February

Edward came ten minutes late and said he'd been earlier. He seemed sad. He started his drawing with two figures – 'a snowman' – looks female with a beard? This was followed by a ghost-like – the snowman. I suggested the 'spirit of someone dead' – 'Yes – the spirit of someone dead' he repeated. Then he drew cowboys and Charlie Chaplin. Charlie Chaplin wasn't right at first and he threw him into the bin. He made two more attempts at Charlie Chaplin which were also cast into the bin. This throwing of drawings into the bin was most unusual. Eventually, he drew the figure in a way that satisfied. He complained that the crayons were no good – 'all blunt'. I suggested using some of the others and if he passed them to me I could sharpen some, or he could sharpen them himself. He continued drawing cowboys and complaining that it was 'no good'. Then he asked for a drink. I asked him to look through the drawings but says he doesn't want to to-day. He agrees to look next week. I say how things seem to be all wrong today. He then begins to talk spontaneously about his dad and how he doesn't come anymore – 'a while ago – a few weeks ago stopped coming'. He asks the staff on the ward to telephone but he doesn't come. 'Dad says he's in a wheelchair' and Edward tells me how he used to go to the canteen with him and he wanted him to stay longer but he has to go to catch his bus. Edward now suggested that 'he couldn't be bothered to come'. I asked about his mother. 'She used to come with him – can't come by herself' 'They lived round the corner past where the flowers are – little flat' he then described the rooms. Very much in touch with his feelings today – I felt – and I had not seen this before. He asks if I could give him some money for the canteen – so he could go and get cigarettes. I said No, and told him what I felt my role was, to help him use the space and materials in here, and I suggested that I didn't think it would help him if I gave him money. He said that was what 'W. did he stole money from the pockets of nurses coats in the nurses home'.

I spoke to the staff again about his wish to see his father. I did think that Edward was preparing himself for his father's death, in the only way possible, given his situation. There is a possibility that his father did not wish to see him. At the beginning of the session, it seems as if, his father, and perhaps his mother as well in the form of the snowman, have already become ghosts. The beard could be a reference to my beard...

July

I spoke about a two-week holiday which was forthcoming. He drew a castle with lots of windows, then ships, a boat, a table and chairs inside a church – 'the preachers chair', he said. Next followed a parrot, a man riding a horse, a giraffe and an elephant sitting down. He also drew a tiger which he said was 'a wild tiger'. I did, despite his words, remark on it not looking fierce. Then there were tanks 'firing at castle', he said. There were cars going into the castle 'that queer fellow – queer bloke' in the car going inside. Two boxers were then drawn in a schematic abstract way. I linked the boxers to the other sportsmen and his thoughts about forming a relationship here with me – in the past – one person having to knock the other person down – perhaps. The iron man with letters on his arms and body followed, he was unable to tell me what the letters were about – he said 'he lights up'. The cars going into the castle, and 'that queer fellow' suggest an unwanted phallic entrance, perhaps the queer bloke who inscribes the letters on the body of the iron man, who then 'lights up'. I was happy to think that the iron man, at this moment, exemplifies the insight that is gained when access to the symbolic realm is possible.

*It could be that Edward at the beginning of this session was referencing a visit to a church possibly a funeral. An exact date for the death of **both** parents is not given in any of the records I had access to, but it seems to have been in March of this year. Edward did not speak about these deaths directly.*

December

Edward began by drawing a house, plus radio, table and chair, followed by boys mostly with baseball caps that were cross-hatched. Sometimes the boys had hands in pockets, others were engaged in activities. There was a boy on scooter, a boy on a bike, a boy 'playing ball', 'holding up a finger', a boy with his 'hands up', one boy on his own, and one boy on a rocking chair who 'can't sit still'. Thinking of my own movements in the session I asked him if he was thinking of me in the session – 'Yes mister'.

When we were looking at the drawing of the radio I asked him if he had a radio at home (thinking here of radio programmes he has referred to, for example, 'Dick Barton' and 'Educating Archie'). He said 'No' he 'went across the road to a place – you know mister – where they have statues with their head cut off – big Jesus on the wall'. Then later said he didn't have a radio because he was 'handicapped' and 'didn't know how to switch it on'. He continued, 'Parents have one – they got a telly – but not for a long time'. He spoke of 'Ena Sharples' dying. I asked are you still handicapped? I then asked what were the things that he couldn't do. Edward said 'Can't do them hand puzzles, can do wooden ones, can't read, can't write properly – tried to learn but can't do it'. I then asked him what his parents thought about his handicap. He then spoke about a film and dynamite and blowing up. I said that it sounds like your parents found it very difficult to think about. 'Yes mister', he replied. I felt I wanted to end on a positive note and I suggested that the two of us in here were like the boys playing together.

The radio suggested to me a mind, that he had been robbed of a mind in some way and that he needed help to switch it on. I wonder now if my asking about the things he couldn't do wasn't after all producing him as a 'handicapped' subject, through the interaction. I may be right about being robbed of a mind, but what is it in interactions and situations that robs the individual of mind? Included in that should be my mind.

Year 6

March

Edward came on time he drew a house, sun, moon, man and woman. The house was drawn between the woman and the man, and the man was seen under the moon and the woman under the sun. Edward said that he thought the moon, which he connected with night, was male, and the sun, he connected with the day, was female. I asked if the couple, the man and the woman, or parents, lived in the house, 'yes', he said. Did he think about his mum and dad still, 'yes', was his reply. Next came some pictures of fighting: a woman was firing guns from a ship at a man in a boat. A bridge and smaller boat were drawn on the back of this composition. It was unusual for Edward to use the back of the sheet of paper.

I asked did mum fight with dad? 'No mister', Edward said. He drew an aeroplane which was being shot down by a boat, there was a door into boat, and another aeroplane 'was landing'. In the next picture an aeroplane was dropping bombs on a boat – 'breaks his leg – kills him – the man in the boat', Edward indicated. The iron man was drawn with a man beside him – he 'grinds things up with his teeth – eats things – smashes up the furniture – the mirror'. 'Out of control' I suggested to Edward. 'The man mends him – the electrics inside', he said. Superman and batman with glasses follow, then Humpty Dumpty sitting on the wall.

I did think that there was a real connection between the parental couple, the guardians of day and night, and the fighting. The real reply to my question is the fighting between the boats, and the fighting between the boat and the aeroplane, and the man who has his legs broken and then is killed by bombs. The imagery presents a violent family where the iron man smashes the mirror. This was the home environment, as suggested by the hospital records. He became quite anxious near the end hurrying to complete more work, to avoid any further comments from me, I felt.

I was puzzled in this session, wondering if I could find a sensitive way of making links between the images and narratives, making something clearer, for him, and for myself. Edward is remembering his parents and home in this session I feel sure. The positive aspect is that the Iron Man is capable of being mended, maybe it requires a superman or batman. In this session, man is associated with the moon and woman with the sun, but in a previous drawing this position was reversed, maybe that tells us something about the parental relationship?

May

Drawings began with profiles of men with hats, (the French Man hat) and the men had jackets and trousers with pockets. He next drew a 'Soldier – pulling out a hand-kerchief'. The 'handkerchief' was not drawn. Humpty Dumpty was drawn next and Edward pointed out that he had arms and legs. The iron man followed, next a tank and man in a car. The iron man, who in this picture has a large hand is 'crushing' the man in the car 'to pieces' – 'when he catches him'. A castle was drawn with the drawbridge up which was manned with armed soldiers. Two full faces followed which represented his mother and his father, smiling. Then a policeman, 'he locks people up', Edward said. He spoke about his father and mother with my encour-agement and he said that they were dead and very briefly described going to his father's funeral, he spoke of the black cars and meeting his parent's neighbours, neighbours who did visit him in hospital. I remarked that it was good that he was able to draw his parents smiling and I suggested that maybe he had some good memories of his parents.

I said that I was wondering about the Iron Man and the castle and I suggested that the iron man attacked the man in the car and was expecting to be attacked in re-turn, reminding him of the castle with drawbridge up. When we came to the police-man I suggested that this could also be connected with the attack of the iron man. Thinking of the iron man smashing furniture and the mirror and influenced by the hospital documents which suggest an earlier difficult relationship with parents, I then suggested that perhaps the iron man's attack was an attack on parents. Edward, unsurprisingly, was not willing to think about my interpretation at this point and left three minutes early, leaving me to reflect on my urgent need to hear something further from Edward about his past.

My interpretation was going too far too quickly, an abrupt move after the good memories of my parents. I may have anticipated that this reported conflictual rela-tion to parents could be thought about. But it looks as if I wanted an acknowledge-ment or a confession in relation to his violent past. The man in the car might well have been the therapist, as included in the hospital reports is Edward throwing stones at cars belonging to the staff.

At this moment in time, I had just become aware that Edward had found a place in a hostel in the community. No date for his leaving had been given to me at this point.

July

Edward came late after a visit to the chiropodist. He drew three faces, tank and car, moon and sun. I reminded Edward that he would be leaving in three weeks (leaving the hospital) and we only had three weeks left. He drew 'the windmill' with a cow-boy outside. I reminded him of the other windmills he had drawn. He responded, 'get pop inside – I've seen one'. I asked about this memory – 'when I was 12' he said. He went with his parents, and I suggested that this was a good memory and I asked if he would remember the sessions – coming here? 'Yes', he replied.

He drew two men in a boat, then a cowboy with something on the top of his hat – 'chopper thrown at him by Indians – has it in his hat when with the Indians', he explained. I understood this as a reference to Edward's need to continue to protect himself. Further drawings followed, a cowboy, donkey man, man in car, two men in boat – 'gold' in boat 'they're taking up the river to a factory'. I point to the guns on the boat and suggest that the gold has to be kept safe – 'it's something that needs looking after' – like the good memories of parents, and maybe memories of here. This was followed by a 'man', 'Humpty Dumpty', a house with 'shed' attached, and the sun with a startled wide-eyed expression.

I seem to want to build on the positive aspects of the windmill which Edward has foregrounded. My feeling is Edward still needs to protect himself and the gold which I like to think of as a therapeutic achievement, an intersubjective achievement.

August

Edward arrived late he told me he had been drinking tea on the ward. It was possible that he had arrived early and returned to the ward. I asked and he said 'Yes' but it felt difficult to be sure of his 'Yes'. I reminded him of the time left. He drew the sun, the moon and a cowboy on the same sheet. I interpreted this as day and night, opposites coming together, the light of the day and the darkness of the night, I suggested that it could relate to the idea of good and bad coming together, and further I proposed that they may have joined together here in Art Therapy. He responded with 'yes mister opposites'. Since he was echoing my words I felt encouraged to try conversation and I then said 'and now the cowboy was leaving town'.

The next drawing was of two cowboys Edward said 'the other cowboy', and I asked about him but he had nothing to say about this. Next were drawn, a policeman, a sheriff, a cowboy, and a postman. A 'cowboy outlaw' with a tall hat and stripes was drawn next. The 'sheriff' was 'going after him'.

I spoke about visiting him in his new home suggesting that I could see how he was 'getting on' – he agreed to this idea. I asked him about his thoughts of leaving – what did he think about it. After a pause he said – 'I don't know how to do that – I don't know how to use the plasticine mister' I suggested 'maybe you don't know how to think about it, it's too difficult, strange, you're not sure what is happening'. He then drew a pirate. I said how the pirate was like the outlaw stealing and the policeman or sheriff was after him. I suggested that we could use the clay next week and I could show him how it could be used, this might help with plasticine.

It's doubtful that Edward appreciated the good and bad coming together, idea. I did not have any real idea of what the Outlaw and the Pirate were indicating, or what kind of narrative might emerge in relation to these characters. In making a more generalised comment about the problem of the plasticine I was closing down the subject. Responding to it more concretely by offering to show him how plasticine could be used was not the right solution either.

August (2) – A Week Later

Ten minutes early and I asked him to wait. I said that I would move the time to next week because of his visit to the hostel and he agreed to meet on Tuesday. I said that I would visit the hostel, once he had settled in, and take a sketchbook along and he seemed to like that idea.

He waited five minutes before starting drawing and drew faces with eyes which had rounded pupils. He referred to the face with round eyes as 'difficult'. A 'donkey camel pony man' emerged from his drawings and then three different types of judges, with different hats or headgear. The next image of a face was labelled 'Tom brown school days' but also 'John Brown'.

Referring to the drawings I reminded him of the 'donkey camel pony man' in the desert drinking water from the tin can. The judge was 'seen in church' he said. He hadn't been before a judge. Maybe he was thinking of his experiences at the funeral. I wondered if 'John Brown' had reminded him of schooldays but he seemed to regard him as a man (maybe he intended the 'John Brown' of the American Civil War – whose body lies 'a mouldering' in the grave?). I suggested leaving was like facing the desert searching for or needing food and water.

I suggested looking at some older work. He agreed to look but said little about it. He named items sometimes and we came across some very aggressive looking iron men as we leafed through the drawings and also men in a boat. I said how the men in the boat related to us on our journey and spoke about the iron men attacking through biting. The teeth were prominent in the drawings. He then asked to do some more drawing – more faces, judges, the donkey man, and a final iron man who 'lights up' and appears to be wired for thought (see Figure 26). He ended the drawing with pirates which I related to all the paper he helped himself to.

Earlier characters or figures appear to be changing. The judges wear different hats and one appears in church. If John Brown does refer to a death, it results according to the hymn, in a 'soul' that 'goes marching on'. Thus John Brown would seem to represent a loss/ending or a parting. The Iron Man changes from a figure with prominent teeth to one who 'lights up'. I restrained myself from mentioning the good and the bad although I did assign a role to the pirates. The amount of paper has always troubled me.

August (3) – Last Session

Edward came on time and chose some very large sheets of paper. He drew faces, 'John Brown' with different hats, but the face was mostly the same, except for a fat face with glasses and no hat. This was followed by, an aeroplane, ship, boat with sail, Humpty Dumpty and two men 'wrestling' (Figure 39). Then he drew, 'baba black sheep', and 'Tom Thumb' with 'pie'. After 15 minutes, he declared 'I've finished' and he asked for a drink. I asked about the hostel – he seemed enthusiastic and he spoke about it being in a village and there were three ladies – he could smoke fags there but he seemed sure his friends would not visit him and that he would not see them again. Instead of acknowledging this loss I attempted to reassure him by repeating that I would visit 'to see how things were going'.

We looked through the drawings and I said that the faces were the same each time but different hats and suggested this might be him in different disguises. I pointed out that the aeroplane had German and English markings. The ship was empty with no portholes or cargo. Humpty Dumpty had arms and legs outstretched and the wall was superimposed on him. I reminded him of all the previous Humpty Dumpty pictures, sometimes falling off the wall and going into pieces – perhaps we were putting together his pieces here, I suggested. The wrestlers did not have arms but this did not bother Edward. I said that maybe he wrestled with my words/ thoughts here just as I wrestled with his drawings trying to understand. Baba black sheep – he remembered the 'Baba black sheep' rhyme and we dwelt on 'one for the master, one for the dame, one for the little boy who lived down the lane' Everybody had something, I observed. Finally, we came to Tom Thumb 'with the pie', he said. I suggested, 'pulling the plum out of the pie', and I reminded him of all the paper and pencils he had helped himself to here over the years. He pointed out that he didn't 'take pencils out' and I agreed and I said 'No' he 'didn't take drawings away' or take anything but 'left everything here'. 'No' he emphasised.

Shortly after this he wanted to go, I thought, maybe I had offended him with my comments on Tom Thumb. There was 15 minutes to go but Edward declared that he was 'finished'. I think we were both relieved... At the end of this session, I shook hands with him and told him that I enjoyed working with him – He shook hands firmly.

I don't know if I used the words 'helped himself to' – this suggests something illegitimate. I could have spoken about the exchange between us in more positive terms, for example he provided me with drawings to look at and think about, whereas I provided him with materials to use and a cup of tea. I was left feeling sad, and wished I could have been more thoughtful in relation to my comments/interpretations and been more in touch with his feelings throughout our time together. It is not Tom Thumb who pulls plums out of pies, it was 'Little Jack Horner', and it was the last line I was thinking of 'What a good boy am I!' (Opie and Opie 1951). Why did I want some agreement from him that he did use a lot of paper and pastels?

December – Follow Up Visit to Hostel

I met Edward at the hostel while I was talking to the manager and waiting in the kitchen. Edward peered through the kitchen window on returning from the shop where he had been to buy cigarettes. He smiled and appeared animated and pleased to see me. He showed me around the lounge and the dining room. I suggested that we could sit down together and he could do some drawing as I had bought a sketchbook along. He agreed to this idea and after we had found somewhere quiet to sit he soon began drawing.

He began with a drawing of a dog which led me to ask if there were animals in the house. He said 'rabbit'. Next he drew 'Superman' – 'he's thinking'. Then came a cowboy with arms raised. This was followed by the Judge and a racing car. I pointed to lever which he named as 'a brake' and then I pointed out a pedal which could have been an accelerator. I suggested that he may be feeling that everything was happening too quickly and he'd like to apply the brakes. An aeroplane was drawn next, and it appeared to be pointed in two directions. Edward then corrected this without any word from me.

Edward drew a man on a boat – 'captain', he said. Next, he drew a 'prisoner'. Humpty Dumpty followed but there was no sign of a wall, and I said it didn't look like he had fallen down. Two boys wrestling were drawn and some cowboys were completed and then the next seven sheets contained the 'seven dwarfs'. Edward carefully counted them. After the dwarfs, he drew a fire engine and two firemen, and a 'house' which became a 'church'. In relation to the last picture, he said, 'It's him Father'.

We surveyed the drawings, and in response, I spoke very briefly about the past and the future, my returning to the hospital and him staying here. This led Edward to want to end the meeting but he was persuaded to stay until we had finished surveying all the drawings. He insisted I take the drawings away 'You keep them'. After that he showed me a rabbit which was kept in a hut in the garden. He explained how he fed it bits of cauliflower and sat and watched it eating. Edward also showed me his room which he liked. He was happily smoking in the laundry room when I left. The hostel manager told me that Edward had taken up woodworking in the workshop.

The significant communication was the drawing and our looking at the rabbit in the garden. I did wonder if Superman thinking was an ironic response to my arrival. He was reluctant to engage in talk about the past or the future. The sequence of dwarf pictures which Edward carefully numbers ends with the Church and finally father, suggests to me some recognition of his having reached a different place, in life. The numbering may substitute for counting of the years in hospital – much more than seven of course. The image of Edward feeding the rabbit stayed with me and I understood this as a positive sign. I was also glad to hear that he had taken up woodworking.

Final Discussion

As can be seen from my reflections on the beginnings of the therapy, to establish regularity in Edward's attendance, it was incumbent on me to assume the authority invested in me as a member of staff, to recognise and accept the power relation as it necessarily existed in the Hospital setting, and work with it. Edward had established for himself a way of living within the institutional demands that sought to shape his existence. When I first met him his life, after breakfast, was a daily wandering, avoiding any prolonged contact with staff he used his minimal use of language to remain inaccessible to interrogation. He was not in the habit of providing any account of himself, and, in his situation, it is unlikely that he could have provided others with an account of himself that could be heard and understood. The ward staff were willing to help me in my disciplinary intervention since they were anxious in relation to his whereabouts.

As well as the disciplinary element there was a material and discursive element which shaped my thinking about the task that Art Therapy in hospital B represented. The mortuary conversion had been designed for observation (see Figure 2, Chapter 3) and I was expected to report on communication with Edward, to assist in team decision-making. Other staff members who had an interest in psychoanalytical approaches to therapeutic interventions and understandings, encouraged me in imagining that I might disclose something of Edward's subjectivity through the establishment of a relationship mediated by the use of art materials, and I wanted to believe that I was capable of developing those empathic sensitivities considered to be central to my role in providing therapeutic support.

But my rational construction of a brief for myself soon began to deteriorate in the face of my emotional response to Edward's greedy consumption of paper, his refusal, or difficulty with speech, and the broken and scattered oil pastels that he left behind after his abrupt departures. I began to feel there was a demand for something I could not supply, and this demand had within in it a demand that I do not demand from him, but simply give. This demand was experienced as a regressive communication that repeats the helplessness of the human subject at the beginning of life. Lacan writes 'The subject has never done anything other than demand, he could not have survived otherwise' (Lacan 1977, p254).

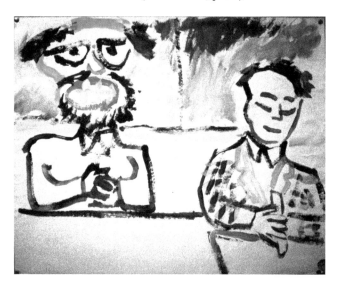

Figure 40 Paint on A2 – the therapist and Edward in the Art Therapy space.

I rapidly executed this painting (Figure 40) at the beginning of the second year of therapy – it was not shared with Edward. I wanted to grasp the strong feelings that inhabited my person after a succession of silent and frustrating sessions with Edward, who cut short my speech by leaving the session early. Edward is on the right of the picture, he appears to be slipping away out of the edge of the frame, he is calmly concentrating on his drawing, giving no indication of having any disturbing feeling whatsoever, whereas the therapist, myself, on the left is wringing his hands and clenching his teeth, barely containing his rage. The teeth, represented through a grid-like form, repeat Edward's strategy when drawing angry faces. There is a stormy black cloud, and something yellow above Edward's head, an external disturbance but nothing, we feel, likely to impact on Edward's apparent serenity.

In Kleinian terms, if Edward *was* giving expression to an unconscious phantasy by leaving his oral aggression within the body and psyche of the therapist, not all the rage that I attempt to express via the painting, should be attributed to Edward's projective capacities. In terms of my conscious desires, I did want some speech to be part of the process, for the relationship to deepen, for reciprocity to develop, hoping for an opportunity to explore, with Edward, the potential symbolic content of the drawings. Secondly, I did have some practical need to conserve sufficient paper and pastels for others to use; but thirdly, more importantly, I felt some pressure to demonstrate that Edward was communicating significantly, through his art making, and verbally, where possible. Quite a large portion of my rage had its origins in my own phantasy and paranoia, a feeling that Edward's response to Art Therapy, if it rendered me redundant, would expose me; it was, I was feeling, a deliberate exhibition of contempt in relation to the rationality of my brief. Consequentially my credentials for being any kind of art therapist would turn out to be fraudulent.

Lacan suggests that to speak is to make a demand, and that the other, the addressee, is expected to respond. Bion (1967, p91) argues that the analyst's insistence on the verbal could be felt as an attack by the patient on '*his* methods of communication' (Bion's italics) thus destroying an important form of contact that enables speech to emerge. But Bion complicates this (op cit p105 & p107) and proposes that an analyst who remains 'balanced' can be seen to present a 'hostile indifference' or if demonstrating understanding can be hated for this, through envy.

I did want to find an intervention that might help Edward tolerate the verbal, even if that verbal element remained minimal. But for Edward drawing *was* communication. He placed his completed drawings on the table quite deliberately in between us, sometimes with a brief 'here y'are', and a quick look towards me. This suggests that he felt I could understand these visual signifiers, and I did treat them as communications, in particular as vehicles for the development of symbolic thought and the transmission of feeling, feelings that could be linked to events in the sessions.

From year 2 Edward began to attend regularly and often remained for the whole session. He became more absorbed in image-making and his absorption excluded me. Edward, I felt, was lost in the imaginary and my speech was irrelevant. My speech was ignored. The sessions were largely filled with silence. When Edward came late, or early, as he sometimes did, he sat down and began drawing whether I was present in the studio or not. The office was immediately next door and Edward would walk past the office door, he would have seen me in the office before entering the studio, but he was not interested in letting me know that he had arrived. My failure to sit and wait in the studio or notice when he arrived was an indication of my inability to keep in contact with him, and this lack of attention and his reaction, could both be regarded as a species of 'hostile indifference', an affect present in the sessions, that we each assigned to the other.

It has to be said that Edward's facial expressions were not easy to read, and his body language was not overtly expressive, and I did struggle to consciously apprehend feeling in the situation. If what I have named, following Bion, as 'hostile indifference' appeared to have an independent existence of its own, how should we think about this?

Williams (2010) seeks to differentiate emotions, and feeling states, which are seen as essentially bodily phenomena, from affect, which goes beyond corporeal embodiment and represents 'a power to affect and be affected' (p246). She argues that affects are a form of encounter and they circulate productively. Affect is always constructed and mediated culturally, and is a force that exceeds the subject. In a parallel approach to affect, Wetherell (2013) emphasises language as an 'affective practice', a 'carrier of affect' which 'enables it to be shared between subjects'. Importantly Wetherell argues that subjects are 'not only constituted through the movement of affect between subjects' but are also 'interpolated' that is recognised and constituted as subjects in 'in social grids of meaning and power' (see Campbell and Pile 2015, p2) in this way subject to the larger social, cultural and political domain. Thinking in this way we might simply regard the 'hostile indifference' as something that belonged to staff/resident relations in the hospital, something replicated in a situation where the staff member is busy in his world, and where the resident seeks to explore interests in *his* world.

In their reading of Freud's case study of Frau Emmy von N., Campbell and Pile op cit, seek to show that the gap between the registration of emotion and affects cannot be simply closed by 'assuming that the words for affects refer to the affects themselves' and that it should be recognised that 'affects emerge between the patient and the doctor, unconsciously', through 'passionate forms' (p18). This view represents a challenge to Wetherell, in that it is proposed that discourse is not sufficient for accessing affect. But neither are affects 'pre-social, uncommunicative, and incapable of finding forms' (p21). Rather words, like symptoms, 'are structured by unconscious processes' and verbalising 'entrains and is entrained by affects' (p18 & p19). Unconscious communication is not 'uni-directional' in the therapeutic setting and Campbell and Pile argue that to achieve understanding it is necessary to 'work with the entanglements between unconscious communication and conscious expression'.

Verbal language is privileged in psychoanalytical practices, from which, alongside other art therapists, I drew theoretical support. The verbal was privileged in the discourses of the hospital, and in fact its presence or absence, and/or deformations, constituted subjects as having, or lacking, capacities. Although I supposed that I was giving proper due to Edward's drawing as *language* and that I had some awareness of its ability to absorb and transport affect, I did not appreciate the entanglements involved, especially the manner in which affect was generated, by non-verbal *and* verbal communication, conscious and unconscious, on the part of the therapist and the resident.

If what I named as a 'hostile indifference' represents an 'affect', that could not be adequately named, I would now say it could be best imagined as Edward's two boxers, but this time as sitting on their corner stools, eyeing each other before the bell sounds for the next round.

In the third year, I began to give more attention to the imagery, perhaps looking unconsciously for 'passionate forms', but also because I felt more confident in Edward's ability to respond robustly to the challenge that my sometimes overt and intrusive demand for speech represented. While I tried to give more attention to my own talk, endeavouring to privately assess how it might be received before speaking, Edward demonstrated his confidence in the setting by continuing to attend, and more hopefully in Session 10 for instance, there was an intimate exchange around fingers and hands indicating the presence of desire and concern. Letters were discussed and this led to my speculation that our relationship could deepen sufficiently to encompass the symbolic. Further, an exploration of protection emerges in relation to the Castle and the Iron Man. 'Protection' was needed in, and for relationships, Edward was telling me.

In year 6 Edward's parents appear in his work and there is some very tentative reflection on past home life. There was some sadness expressed in his drawings which included tears. After giving an account of the Iron Man's aggression in the home environment he expresses a hope that the Iron Man can be mended by having his electrics inside sorted. The radio being in the Iron Man's stomach suggests that it is a feeling, or affect, that needs to be thought, and the switch on the side of the Iron Man indicates a need for external intervention to help with thinking.

In Session 34 Edward expresses anxiety in relation to leaving the hospital and after surveying some previous work, we look at orally aggressive Iron Men. He ended the session with a drawing of the Iron Man and a pirate. The Iron Man is wired across his head, wired for thinking (see Figure 26).

I regard the story of the Iron Man as encapsulating a very positive development. In Edward's story the Iron Man gradually moderates his oral aggression, the farmer teaches him to keep time, and he is able to communicate with the house via the telephone, he listens, and he becomes wired for thinking.

I don't know if Edward ever had access to Ted Hughes' (1968) story of the Iron Man, published in 1968, but Edward's story does resonate with Hughes' account. Hughes' story begins with the Iron Man falling off the cliff, and falling into pieces. The pieces are reconnected through the coming together of the eye and the hand. Iron Man is then able to return to the sea. This is the first appearance. Iron Man later returns from the sea and he exhibits a fantastic appetite for metal. Hogarth, a small boy, helps to trap the Iron Man with iron bait, so that he can be buried. When

Iron Man eventually escapes his earthly trap Hogarth talks to him and leads him to a scrap heap, and befriends him. The story ends with Iron Man saving the world from an alien bat-dragon. This entailed Iron Man thinking and enduring a tortuous melting. Essentially Iron Man's heroic life is a trial. He satisfies his inordinate hunger, for metal, as he learns, with the help of Hogarth, to relate. It is thinking, bodily suffering and feeling that is his destiny.

In the Kleinian account of infancy there is 'an oral-sadistic and anal sadistic expression of destructive impulses, operative from the beginning of life' (Klein 1957, p176). In contrast, she also suggests that for the new-born infant, there arises a more positive innate feeling 'that there exists outside him something that will give him all he needs and desires' (p179). Klein goes on to say that 'unavoidable grievances, reinforce the innate conflict between love and hate' (p180) and that there is a longing for unity and for 'constant evidence of the mother's love' (p179). Is this what Edward demands? Bion was concerned to quantify, or qualify, the inordinate need his patients exhibited, and he has written 'the patient's problem may arise not from his greed for 'the breast'', but 'from his greed for what he considers the world is able to yield to him' (Bion 1967, p139). Klein's account fits closely the Iron Man's career, as supplied by Edward and, in part, by Hughes. But in Hughes account of the Iron Man, he is divorced from community, an alien which the community attempts to bury alive, and it is a recognition of his value to the community that positively ends the story.

Edward was placed in a psychiatric hospital at the age of 13. He was effectively abandoned by his parents who did not want Edward to return to the home environment. They were fearful, they wanted their new address to be kept secret from him, and they felt that Edward should be locked in at night.

According to Goffman (1961) admittance to the psychiatric hospital involves the use of a 'betrayal tunnel'. We could expect that Edward would experience his Next of Kin, his guardians, whom ordinarily he may have turned to for help, to have betrayed him (Goffman 1961, p131, Note 20). Once admitted Edward's abandonment is more or less complete. He is captive and has lost all his previous relationships and supports. He may try to start again with his parents but if they are determined to leave him in the hospital then he has to try to reconstruct his sense of self from an entirely new set of circumstances. Edward's offense would become a 'social fact' (p130). We do not know what information may have been available to Edward but he would surely become aware of the 'coalition that has been formed against him' (p129). Like Ted Hughes' Iron Man he is effectively buried. He cannot return to the home environment.

Schaverien (2015) writing about the Boarding School experience of her clients, seen in analytical psychotherapy, describes the shock of abandonment and the bereavement that follows entry into the school. There is homesickness, resulting from the loss of relationships and the loss of familiar and comforting surrounds, and subsequently, there is grief, Schaverien tells us. Goffman points out that there are 'mortifying restrictions' that accompany 'communal living' (Goffman 1961, p137). Schaverien points out that in being captive there is regimentation, and a lack of privacy, and she reports that an insulating shell of toughness is often developed, 'armoured his feelings are hidden even from himself' (p182), a mental state reminding us of the Iron Man, as he first appears in Edward's drawing.

In the setting of the total Institution, Hospital B, how does the intersubjective form of self-reflection get going? Sartre's focus on seeing and being seen could be helpful here. Sartre makes use of Hegel in his account of 'Being-for-others'. He writes 'the primary fact is the plurality of conscious-nesses' which is 'realized in the form of a double, reciprocal relation of exclusion'. 'The very fact of being me' excludes the other. The other 'excludes me by being himself' (Sartre 1956, p319). Encountering the other, and thereby becoming aware of myself, is to apprehend myself as seen. To be seen is to be aware of being in 'the midst of the world, as a thing among things, with properties and determinations that I am without having chosen them' (see Zahavi 2008, p95). This experience, I would suggest, is amplified in the 'Total Institution' where subjects are objectified.

Sartre had a particular interest in shame and he imagines himself jealously peering through a key hole when suddenly he hears footsteps in the hall. This situation which brings with it the realization that somebody maybe looking at him results in an 'irruption of the self' he now sees himself because somebody sees him. Sartre writes 'I am for myself only as I am a pure reference to the Other' Shame according to Sartre is shame of self: 'it is the *recognition* of the fact that I am indeed that object which the Other is looking at and judging' (p350, Sartre's emphasis).

Shame we can imagine as a recurrent experience for Edward throughout his institutional life, and shame was certainly present for Edward in the Art Psychotherapy. If Sartre is right, it is because he was seen, seen to be judged. The repetition of the 'Judge' figure in the drawings is, I would argue, related to the repetitive experience of being seen and objectified. I myself experienced shame when Edward scolded me for interfering in the production of his drawings, and when I failed to notice his entry into the art room. My shame was related to the institutional demand, to bring Edward into relationship with the staff, so that he might provide a communication that would endorse the institutions raison d'etre. In this process, I wanted Art Therapy to be seen as a significant intervention.

Both, this phenomenological and philosophical literature, and Kleinian literature, aim at unearthing fundamental beginnings. Both literatures are productive in providing propositions that enable Psychotherapeutic practices to be interrogated and shaped. Sartre and Klein, you might say, in response, are worlds apart. Certainly Sartre would not endorse Klein's Freudian metapsychology and emphasis on instinct, and we can imagine Klein criticising Sartre for his refusal to recognise the unconscious dimension of mental activity. But both give an emphasis to the conflictual in the intersubjective creation of relationship – Klein through her emphasis on envy, Sartre through his foregrounding of shame. Envy is contrasted in Klein by the infant's desire for unity and the development of gratitude. Sartre seeks to demonstrate that solidarity is achieved through recognition and reciprocity. It is in relation to the 'Third', the totality that shapes 'Us', the dyad or the group, that shame is mitigated, I want to suggest, despite the negative effects of institutional power.

The 'Third' enabled Edward and me to persevere with our attempts at relating and communicating over time. Time and consistency allowed Edward to tolerate my use of language, and it allowed me to appreciate his production of imagery, imagery that enabled symbolic communication to emerge and affect to be processed so that we both might gain an appreciation of the other. Recognition was Edward's gain from Art Therapy, when reciprocity became possible, and where together we could both overcome contestation.

This thinking about recognition, I want to develop in the next inconclusive concluding chapter.

References

Atkinson, D. 2002. *Art in Education – Identity and Practice*. Kluwer Academic Publishers, Dordrecht, Boston, London.

Bion, W. F. 1967. *Second Thoughts*. William Heinemann Medical Books Ltd. Reprinted by H. Karnac (Books) Ltd., 1993, London.

Campbell, J. & Pile, S. 2015. Passionate Forms and the Problem of Subjectivity: Freud, Frau Emmy Von N. and the Unconscious Communication of Affect, *Subjectivity* 8(1): 1–24.

Goffman, E. 1961. *Asylums – Essays on the Social Situation of Mental Patients and Other Inmates*. Penguin Books, London.

Hughes, T. 1968. *The Iron Man Illustrated: Andrew Davidson*. Faber and Faber Ltd., London.

Klein, M. 1957. Envy and Gratitude. Chapter 10 pp 176–235 In: *Envy and Gratitude and Other Works 1946–1963*. Virago Press Ltd., London.

Lacan, J. 1977. Chapter 7 - The direction of the treatment and the principles of its power pp 226–280 In: *Jacques Lacan Ecrits a Selection Trans: Sheridan, A*. Routledge, London.

Opie, J. & Opie, P. (Eds.) 1951. *The Oxford Dictionary of Nursery Rhymes*. Oxford at the Clarendon Press, London, Glasgow, New York, Toronto, Melbourne, Wellington, Bombay, Calcutta, Madras, Cape Town.

Sartre, J. P. 1956. *Being and Nothingness*. Barnes, H. E. (Trans.). Washington Square Press – Pocket Books, New York, London, Toronto, Sydney, Tokyo, Singapore.

Schaverien, J. 2015. *Boarding School Syndrome – The Psychological Trauma of the 'Privileged' Child*. Routledge, Hove, East Sussex, New York.

Van Sommers, P. 1984. *Drawing and Cognition – Descriptive and Experimental Studies of Graphic Production Processes*. Cambridge University Press, London, New York, New Rochelle, Melbourne, Sydney.

Wetherell, M. 2013. Affect and Discourse – What's the Problem? From Affect as Excess to Affective/Discursive Practice, *Subjectivity* 6(4): 349–368.

Williams, C. 2010. Affective Processes Without a Subject: Rethinking the Relation Between Subjectivity and Affect with Spinoza, *Subjectivity* 3(3): 245–262.

Wollheim, R. 1984. *The Thread of Life*. Cambridge University Press, Cambridge, London, New York, New Rochelle, Melbourne, Sydney.

Zahavi, D. 2008. *Subjectivity and Selfhood – Investigating the First-Person Perspective*. MIT Press, Cambridge, London.

Conclusion

Recognition

Discourses, medical and psychological, present impairment as a natural malformation, as a body that is lacking from the beginning, or it has become damaged in some respect. Essentially the individual is seen as 'defective', to use the older more pejorative term. In the case of the Learning Disabled, there is an identified, inferred or hypothesised, neurological malformation or damage, which brings the mind into question. Whatever is the result of the impairment, whether it leads to an adaptation or results in difficulties with particular tasks, in making a diagnosis, a disability is socially constructed, and it is productive of a subject whose participation in community life is consequentially restricted.

Amy and Edward were obliged to join a 'confused family of "abnormals"' (Foucault 2000) that, from the turn of the 20th century to 1930s, generated a collective fear of degeneration expressed as a demand for incarceration and separation, which was enacted through Governmental Policy and legislation in Britain. Not all those in a position of power who might shape governmental policy in respect of the disabled, and others, were in favour of this response, but somehow those children, adolescents and adults, who were regarded as deficient in mind, were, in particular, thought to represent a 'moral' danger to the population at large. Abnormals were seen as failing to assume, or perform their duties according to the 'position in life' to which they were born (Tredgold 1908). Consequentially people, especially from those poorer sections of the working classes which had become destitute, suffered catastrophic injustices. Amy was resident in an educational institution from the age of 13 and admitted to Hospital B at the age of 17 years, in 1949. Edward was admitted to a large Psychiatric hospital at age 13, and three years later to Hospital B, in 1955. Amy died in Hospital B 47 years later. Edward was moved to a hostel in the community after living in Hospital B for 40 years.

How does an incarcerated subject who has no legal redress, but is subject to Medical and institutional authority, gain recognition from the other? I implied in the Summary of Chapter 5 that 'recognition' was made possible in Art Therapy through time and consistency, where a necessary reciprocity could emerge which facilitates intersubjective appreciation of the other, and where the therapeutic dyad finds some support from a third larger Other (the setting). I still want to hold to this view but what is this recognition that I referred to? Some theory is necessary here.

DOI: 10.4324/9781003360056-7

In this speculative conclusion, I will be drawing on Butler's reflections on Hegel's Phenomenology of the Spirit and Sartre's use of Hegel. I have made use of Innwood's Hegel Dictionary and Hegel himself, but my intention is to try to keep the philosophy and theory brief. I am interested in disclosing recognition in its situated aspect, where that is possible.

Butler views Hegel's Phenomenology as a Bildungsroman, a narrative that provides us with a fictional account of a consciousness journeying towards self-awareness. Within this, a 'strategy for appropriating philosophical truth' is disclosed. There is a deliberate comedy of failure in this narrative Butler suggests, but she argues that Hegel's provisional scenes, 'the stage of self-certainty, the struggle for recognition, the dialectic of lord and bondsman, are instructive fictions' (Butler1999, p21). Recognition in Hegel's presentation of recognition as 'Anerkennung' is more than 'simply the intellectual identification of a thing or person' but includes within it acknowledgement. It is self-consciousness which seeks recognition and with it an acknowledgement. According to Innwood's account of Hegel's thinking, 'Self-consciousness's first attempt to establish itself is to satisfy its desire by consuming one object after another'. But recognition/acknowledgement requires reflection, which comes from another, 'a self on a par with one's own self'. To make use of 'I' 'requires the use of use of "he/she" as well as of "it"' (Innwood 1995, p246 & p247).

Butler emphasises that desire is the 'logical motor' of the Phenomenology, desire as 'embodied' and situated, and she argues that Hegel's drama illustrates the operative force of desire, seen as sequential; that is, 'consuming desire, desire for recognition, desire for another's desire' (Butler, 1999 p43). Sartre observes, following Hegel, that 'the road of interiority passes through the Other'. I can 'be an object for myself only over there in the Other' and this indicates that I must 'obtain from the Other *recognition* of my being' (Sartre, 1956 p320, Sartre's emphasis). Here we can see, according to Hegel's notion of recognition, recognition emerges from desire and emerges in subjectivity and intersubjectivity.

In Chapter 2 I briefly described my research with 'Alfred' (p39) a young man who enjoyed painting. Alfred was diagnosed as having a 'childhood psychosis' when admitted to Hospital B and he lived in 'K' ward. 'K' ward provided a residence for young men, from late teens to mid-thirties, who experienced difficulties in communication and social interaction. In Alfred's ward, I also met 'Robert'. Alfred and Robert were not able to speak and both were regarded as having severe learning disabilities. It was difficult for these young men to gain admittance to day care in the hospital, mostly because their behaviour was thought to be very 'challenging', and few staff were willing to risk interaction with them.

'K' ward was sparsely furnished; some large wedge-like foam shapes, covered in a brightly coloured plastic vinyl, were scattered around the perimeter of the day room. In the dining room, there were chairs and tables. On one side of the day room were tall windows, and the opposite walls were bare. At the back of the ward, through the dining room and dormitory, was a yard surrounded by high fences. Usually the dining room and the yard were only accessible by the residents when escorted by staff.

In the corner of the day room was the nurses' office which was surrounded by glass windows allowing for observation of the day room, where residents sat or lounged and sometimes paced around the perimeter, or rocked themselves from a standing position. There was some recognition within hospital B that this environment was impoverished, and a new younger Psychiatrist was endeavouring to improve the environment and find therapeutic support for the residents, from whatever the Hospital could provide. I agreed to give help where I could.

Robert was over six foot tall and broad, physically intact, and handsome. On my first visit to the ward, I entered via the main door off a corridor, after agreeing a time with the nurses. Closing the door behind me I took about three paces towards the opposite end of the day room where the nurses' office was situated when Robert came through the dining room door and charged. He ran across the day room towards me making a loud screaming noise, his eyes fixed on my face. I remained still and endeavoured to maintain, as far as possible, a steady gaze, in response to this frightening behaviour. The main idea was not to panic, but this was not a considered strategy rather the moment itself generated a response, retreat did not seem possible, and you could consider my lack of movement as the product of a successful petrification. Robert stopped at about 18 inches from me, his face then broke into laughter. As Robert reached me, two nurses ran towards us. Robert then deftly evaded the nurses and made his way quickly back into the dining area.

Robert had made his presence known to me and I was obliged to recognise my limitations, and something of his potential power. We could regard Robert's behaviour as agonistic display, for the nurses and for the stranger, an assertion of power and status, a claim for territory; this form of ethological analysis and interpretation might be regarded as sufficient explanation for this impressive performance.

Sartre, in his later work, wanted to show in detail how the individual is related to the larger whole, to situations, to groups, ensembles and, ambitiously, the totality as it is manifest in history. In 'Search for a Method', he stresses signifying practices that reference future and absent objects, present in our material environments. Sartre explains that when his 'companion … starts towards the window' he understands 'his gesture in terms of the material situation in which' they are 'both' located. 'He is going "to let in some air"' (Sartre 1968, p153). He stresses 'Within the room, doors and windows are never entirely passive realities; the work of other people has given to them their meaning, has made out of them instruments, possibilities *for an other* (any other)'. Sartre's companion reveals to him 'the practical field' and allows him to 'comprehend the enterprise', his companion *unifies* the room, and the room defines his conduct' (p153 & p154, Sartre's emphasis). Sartre argues that all objects are signs: 'By themselves they indicate their use and scarcely mask the real project of those who have made them such *for us* and who address us through them' (p155, Sartre's emphasis). Sartre refers to this equipment as the 'practico-inert'.

In the hospital, both residents and staff experience imposed subjectivities, ordered identities and possibilities, in relation to action and encounters with others. This is supported by the material situation, in the geography of the hospital grounds, in the buildings, their interior organisation and equipment.

In ward K, the day room is the usual place for residents. The minimally functioning furniture, and lack of stimulation in terms of décor, signals an absence of mind, it is an arena for self-stimulation and bodily performance. The dining room is designed for eating at a table in the presence of staff, the yard for exercise under supervision. The nurses' office is designed for administration surveillance and secure retreat. It was also a space in which a group solidarity could be developed. The nurses reported to me that they often allowed Robert to retire to the dining room. Were he to be confined to the day room he would antagonise other residents; in order, the nursing staff suggested, to amuse himself. The day room and the dining room were Robert's domain, and I was a stranger who was obliged to navigate this environment by seeking the nurses' assistance. Robert's performance becomes paradigmatic, communicating that social interaction, in this setting, with this group of residents, entails difficulties. For sure, Robert's performance was a transmission of feeling. I would judge it to be related to a larger affect 'circulating productively' (Williams 2010) amongst the staff, including, myself the art therapist, and the other residents present in the day room, at that brief, but elevated, moment.

But Robert was knowing in the situation, he was self-aware, and his laughter suggested that he could calculate the other's response to his movements and sounds, and gain enjoyment from his performance, gain an affirmation of sorts. Robert, as an individual, was surely making claims for his achievement, and it is 'for that *being-there* that I demand rights' (Sartre 1956, p324). He is demanding an acknowledgement, and in his making of that claim, we are assuming that desire is at work and a form of reciprocity is required, that is, acknowledgement from the other. Butler, explicating Hegel, writes that desire (in Hegel) is implicit in the transition between consciousness and self-consciousness which 'emerges as a kind of knowing that is at once a mode of becoming; it is suffered, dramatized, enacted' (Butler 1999, p28). We learn later that desire is a desire for 'Life', but, in the beginning at least, the subject who desires 'this proper object of desire' is 'incapable of living, so that desire is mixed with pathos'. considered as 'an initial stage of self-consciousness, the subject is wise to Life without being "of" it' (Butler 1999, p36). This might be another way of thinking about Robert.

The desire for 'Life' was certainly present in Amy and Edward, and, I would judge, sufficient self-consciousness to be wise to 'Life'. If, 'being "of" it' means participating in Life, participation might well be limited and problematic in an institutional setting which identifies you as a subject marked by a deficiency.

Amy volunteered herself for Art Therapy. She was interested in making a new relationship, and in her first two sessions, she presents herself as ordinary, by asserting her independence of thought, and by making comparisons between herself and others. In her initial move to gaining recognition, she is anxious in relation to the possible murderous motives of the therapist, and she wants assurance that the relationship, should it develop, will have within it some predictable reciprocity. Obtaining recognition entails conflict, and since recognition is often 'unequal and insufficient', a reciprocity is needed. 'The value of the Other's recognition of me depends on the value of my recognition of the Other' (Sartre 1956, p320).

There is an awareness that the situation requires work and desire but Amy needs the 'token' of tea, along with regularity, as a guarantee of commitment on the part of the Therapist (myself). The staff are not reliable, and they take Bank Holidays off and are capable of cruelty. 'Bullet' is the exemplar in relation to staff, and 'Bullet' has 'a brick swinging in her heart'. Furthermore, the staff act illegally. Amy knows – 'I know you're staff aren't you'. She knows when I am 'Being bossy' and I have a 'devil inside', just like her brother and herself. Amy experiences my abandonment of her when I cancel a session at short notice and do not offer an alternative time, and she witnesses me being 'cruel' to Barry, leaving him out in the cold. The hate and fear of murderous feelings, expressed in the Jekyll and Hyde image, belongs as much to me as it does to Amy.

Reciprocity *is* difficult, but we have to listen to each other's point of view, otherwise, the radio/mind is messed up (see Session 38). This suggests the self-consciousness of 'Scepticism' in the Phenomenology where the 'negativity of free self-consciousness comes to know itself in the many and varied forms of life as a real negativity'. It can become 'like the squabbling of self-willed children' (Hegel 1977, p123, para 202 & p126, para 205). Amy is tempted to promote fighting between her male friends, and between me and Michel, who was providing Amy with some Counselling. She remembers her parents fighting and remembers experiencing her mothers' murderous rage. We fight together around lateness and my wish to maintain a regularity in our work together, but it is important that Amy is assured that I can, at least try to gain *some* understanding of how it feels to be a resident in hospital B, in that position where she is insulted, abused and called a 'Mental Defective'. If my recognition of her is to be valued it becomes vital that she interrogates my response to her pain. Thus Amy moves towards the '*unhappy, inwardly disrupted* consciousness' a consciousness 'having present in the one consciousness the other also' (Hegel 1977, p126, para 207, emphasis in original) – Precisely the position of Dr Jekyll.

Edward, in the beginning, engages in Art Therapy confidently, producing drawing and naming the content of his imagery, the ship going into the harbour, bridges, the castle and houses, and a man playing a drum. There is a possibility of relationship, implied, in his imagery, a coming home, but also a suggestion of future conflict, hinted by the drummer and the castle. He appears to appreciate the acknowledgement that this imagery was able to generate when shared with me, the stranger, the new art therapist. But, perhaps because he feels that it is a test or an examination of some sort, he does not want to engage in any prolonged verbal interaction and he is not sure that he wishes to revisit the situation a second time. Thereafter, for much of the first year, he attends briefly for 15 minutes, or 10 minutes and then hurries away when I begin to speak.

I do make a demand for a continuous and regular engagement in Art Therapy. I question his absence from the department and I use my authority as a member of staff to ensure a regular attendance. Edward was thus obliged to make some accommodations to institutional processes and negotiate another relationship within the hospital that was asymmetrical in terms of power.

Edward dutifully attends regularly in the second year, and he produces a mountainous amount of drawings, which he wants to leave with the art therapist. This replicates the Lordship and Bondsman relation that Hegel describes, beginning para 178, p111, in the Phenomenology. He is happy for the therapist to view his products but he ensures that the verbal exchanges are kept to a minimum, leaving abruptly when there is too much in the way of speech. Production takes place in silence, apart from some labelling of imagery. Edward tells me about the man (in a film) caught up by the mechanism in a Windmill, going round and round – this is his anxiety.

If Edward feels hopelessly trapped in this servile relationship, it does nevertheless develop. Hegel describes the bondsman as fearful of the Lord at the beginning, experiencing a 'dread' where the 'solid and stable has been shaken to its foundations' (Hegel 1977, p117, para 194) but achieving a self-consciousness through the 'Work' which 'forms and shapes the thing', where the 'object has independence'. Hegel proposes; 'It is in this way, therefore, that consciousness, *qua* worker, comes to see in the independent being [of the object] its *own* independence' (para 195, p118, emphasis in original).

In year 2 my demand for speech increases. I seem to believe that Edward could give a full account of himself, an account that might meet the demands of the institution. Speech would more significantly indicate a recognition and I would then be able to recognise my notion of self in and through my relationship with Edward. However; 'What really confronts' the Lord in the Bondsman is 'not an independent consciousness, but a dependent one' and he (the Lord) is therefore uncertain of his '*being-for-self* as the truth of himself' (Hegel 1977, para 192, p117). My desire to limit the amount of materials that Edward used should be read as an attempt to escape Edward's dependency, and my dependency on Edward.

Edward became more absorbed in his making and appears to retreat into a private imaginary space, just as I retreat into my silence, and the office at times. Each in his own domain 'The other' becomes 'a connected system of experiences out of reach' (Sartre 1956, p310). Edward gains confidence in spontaneously relating in year 3. He speaks of the need for protection against others. Others I understand as principally being the staff. I began to see my role as keeping good time and remaining attentive, giving proper attention to the imagery in the drawings, their sequential presentation and Edward's sparse comments. I also learned that I had to tolerate Edward's excessive use of the materials the hospital supplied.

The 'boxers' suggest a recognition of the competitive nature of our relationship. Differences are present, for example, in the drawing of the drivers going in different directions, although other drawings of couples do often illustrate unity. The Iron Man does find that his mind can be switched on and the Farmer does help him to keep time. Time here in the context of the farm suggests growth.

You could say, using Sartre's words, that to establish reciprocity it was necessary for Edward and myself to move from a '*frontal* opposition' towards 'an oblique interdependence' (Sartre 1956, p331, author's emphasis). This 'interdependence' is achieved through the mediation of Art Materials, and oddly, supported by the shared situation, by the hospital's institutional practices to which we were both subject, albeit differentially.

What reading and thinking have indicated is that a failure to install a dyadic relation that includes 'interdependence' is likely to result in failure of recognition, reciprocity will decay and self-consciousness suffer. To establish a productive dyadic relation, there must be a persistence in the interaction over time, so that desire can move relations towards another future, where the possibility of communication, verbal and non-verbal, can emerge, where affect is held and utilised, so that self-consciousness can find self-consciousness in the other. In the drama both protagonists must find their self-consciousness mirrored and enhanced in the other. Both, the art therapist (myself) and the residents (Amy and Edward) were obliged to learn from the other, each discovering themselves in a process where self-awareness was continuously on the move. For this precarious practice, self and other must find some support from the third Other, the material, cultural and social world of the many others to which both members of the dyad are enchained.

References

Butler, J. 1999. *Subjects of Desire – Hegelian Reflections in Twentieth-Century France – Reprint Edition.* Columbia University Press, New York.

Foucault, M. 2000. The Abnormals In: Rabinow, P. (Ed.) and Hurley, R. et al. (Trans.) *Ethics Subjectivity and Truth – Essential Works of Foucault 1954–1984.* Penguin Books. London, New York, Victoria Australia, Ontario Canada, New Delhi, Albany New Zealand, Rosebank South Africa, pp. 51–57.

Hegel, G. W. F. 1977. *Phenomenology of Spirit.* Miller, A. V. with Analysis of the Text and Foreword Findlay, J. N. (Trans.). Oxford University Press, Oxford, London, Glasgow, New York, Toronto, Melbourne, Wellington.

Innwood, M. 1995. *A Hegel Dictionary (Paperback Reprint).* Basil Blackwell Ltd, Oxford, Cambridge.

Sartre, J. P. 1956. *Being and Nothingness.* Barnes, H. E. (Trans.). Washington Square Press, Pocket Books, New York, London, Toronto, Sydney, Tokyo, Singapore.

Sartre, J. P. 1968. *Search for a Method.* Barnes, H. E. (Trans.). Vintage Books, a Division of Random House, New York.

Tredgold, A. F. 1908. *Mental Deficiency (Amentia).* Bailliere, Tindall & Cox, Covent Garden, London. Digitized by the Internet Archive in 2016. https://archive.org/details/b28047667 – accessed 08.08.22.

Williams, C. 2010. Affective Processes Without a Subject: Rethinking the Relation Between Subjectivity and Affect with Spinoza, *Subjectivity* 3(3): 245–262.

Index

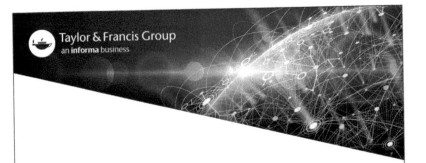